Yoga
and
the Athlete

by Ian Jackson

Published by

World Publications

BOOK OF THE MONTH NO. 45
March, 1975

Copyright © 1975 by RUNNER'S WORLD MAGAZINE

Library of Congress Catalog Card Number: 75-281
ISBN — 0-89037-055-9

World Publications, Box 366, Mountain View, CA 94040

Contents

Foreword

Five minutes after I met Ian Jackson for the first time, he accused me of being a philosopher. I immediately liked the man after an opening like this, even if his analysis was off-base.

My simple-minded definition of a philosopher is one with a gift for seeing common things in uncommon ways. In writing the slim pamphlet called *Long Slow Distance—The Humane Way to Train,* I'd only reported in common language the common things that had happened to me in running. Much as I'd like to, I can't take credit for any original or startling insights.

Ian read the booklet. He read more into it than was on the pages. In fact, any uncommon ideas that came from it were of his and other readers' own making.

Ian Scott Jackson might shake off the label himself, but he's something of a philosopher. When we think of philosophers, we picture hollow-eyed, long-faced men in black coats, looking down on the murky world from a safe distance. Ian isn't like that, he's a thinker for sure, a deep thinker with a talent for cutting through the fluff to the heart of a matter.

But he's more than that. He's a doer—a restless searcher, an experimenter using his own body and mind as a laboratory. He's a bright-eyed, smiling optimist who invests 200% of himself in the passion of the moment.

When I met Ian several years ago, he was nominally a graduate student in English at the University of California, Berkeley. Most of his energy, though, was going into his running. He was running 15-20 miles a day, many of those miles at near-five-minute pace.

Before that, he told me, he'd been a swimmer. He never competed, yet he thrashed out hundreds of laps a week with the UC team. Before that, there had been surfing (he'd dropped out of school to go to Hawaii, to find the biggest waves), an unhappy period of college cross-country racing, skin-diving and spear fishing, soccer (he now edits *Soccer World* magazine) and who knows what else.

In the pre-running period of his life, Ian also experimented with mind-bending drugs and self-hypnosis, was caught stowing away on a ship to Australia, was nearly killed in an auto accident in California and on the coral by a Hawaiian wave.

The running gave Ian an anchor which he'd lacked for a long time, and he held so tightly to it that it almost pulled him down. He went the familiar route of runners who overwork: first to chronic fatigue, then chronic injury.

The search for a way out of these led him on new crusades. Regular readers of *Runner's World* and the booklets will know the direction by the stories Ian has left behind: applications of Hans Selye's stress theories to athletics, natural foods and fasting, and yoga.

All of this wouldn't mean much if Ian simply jumped from one activity to another, dropping the old as he adopted the new. He wouldn't know any more about himself than do the millions of people who ride the waves of fad.

What makes Ian different is that he holds onto the best strands of his experience and ties them to the activity of the moment. This gives his ideas growing strength as they evolve.

Yoga is his current passion (and almost surely not his final one). The devotion to running which once took him to a 2:33 marathon and the dietary discipline which took him down to 116 pounds have moderated. His running and eating habits have found more comfortable places in his lifestyle, as will yoga. Yoga is a philosophy of unity and balance. From the threads of his own diverse background, he is pulling together a unified, balanced philosophy of self-discovery.

Ian is the first person to see clearly the connection between two apparent opposites, yoga and athletics. The popular view of yoga is of malnourished Indians contemplating their navels for hours as they sit contorted like pretzels. What does this have to do with the physical explosiveness of sports and games?

Everything, Ian says. Yoga is deceptively athletic in its physical demands, and it has a lot to teach athletes about physical and psychological flexibility and sensitivity.

Don't let the Sanskrit words scare you away. Yoga isn't as exotic as it sounds. It's simply a way to learn your limitations, your edges. It's stretching without struggling. By repeatedly playing inside the edge of stretch but not fighting past it into pain, you gradually extend your limits.

Awareness in playing your own edges is the essence of yoga. It's also the essence of sound athletic training and healthful living. You don't have to adopt Ian Jackson's entire yoga routine to realize the worth of this philosophy.

—**Joe Henderson**

1 Where I Was or Why

The journey to awareness started in darkness. I held the spear-gun between my knees, and stared at the spearhead as it glistened in the sun. I narrowed my eyes and let the bright sharp edges melt into the sun-glints off the sea. The brilliant blue haze was broken by flashing shadows from passing cars. We had been waiting an eternity. When would the traffic give us space to make our turn?

We never had a chance. We were hit from behind, right into the path of the oncoming cars. Crashes and counter-crashes jumbled in on themselves in fierce density, endlessly. By the time our car spun to the shoulder, it had been battered five times.

My parents were crumpled in the front, broken-backed. I was lying across the rear seat, unconscious. The spearhead had dipped in-to the corner of my eye, bringing up blood. It streamed down the silver shaft and oozed over the black neoprene of my wet suit. But I wasn't there to watch its growing stain. I was in darkness.

For two weeks I was in darkness. Then I ventured out into nightmare.

Lukewarm lights. White-robed ghosts swirling around me. A gloved hand with a glinting needle. Strong arms holding me down. I struggled desperately, until my panic faded back into darkness.

When my eyes next opened, I was in a strange bed in a strange room. A nurse was sitting next to me. She looked at me coldly, then walked out without saying a word. There was no one to tell me where I was or why.

"No more skin diving, "said the doctor when he was giving me a final examination, months later. "You suffered a massive brain bruise from being thrown against the roof of the car. It seems to have gone down completely. But we didn't expect you to pull through and we don't want to take any chances now. Breath-holding is out. Your brain needs all the oxygen it can get. "

The doctor had spoken; he had sentenced me.

"But what can I do if I'm not supposed to go diving anymore?"

"If you don't have any symptoms for a couple of years, you can go diving again. In the meantime, there are plenty of sports you can try. I understand you are a runner. There's nothing wrong with running. In fact, you probably owe your life to it. Just keep on running. It'll keep you in good health."

But running was a sport at school, and because it was so closely connected with school it was somehow tainted from the start. It offered a ready-made identity—"He runs cross-country and track"— which could bring self-respect and respect from others. But it didn't offer a way for me to make my own identity, as skin-diving did. There were no coaches and teams and workouts and meets with skin-diving. Just me and the sea and the excitement of hunting fish and lobster and abalone. With skin diving forbidden, it was inevitable that I would turn to surfing.

The bare land around our house was like hard-baked adobe. The summer after the accident, I spent the morning hours hacking away at it, cutting out patio areas, preparing drainage with sand and gravel, and laying out bricks and paving stone. It helped rebuild my health and it earned me enought money for a surfboard.

At high noon, when the southern California sun turned fierce, I would drop my tools and run down to the beach. My surf heroes were two college men from Arizona. They could barely stand up and turn their boards, but I didn't know any better and, besides, they let me use a board when they came in to rest. They would wave at me when they wanted to go out again. I got pretty good at playing on the edge of innocently not noticing their signals and willfully ignoring them.

"Here's your board, Fred," I'd say. "Thank you very much for letting me use it. How long do you plan to be out this time?"

He'd take it under his arm, crinkle his eyes as he pretended to assess the surf, and answer me in a tone of flat indifference.

"Oh, I guess maybe an hour or two, depending on how I feel."

"Fred, I'm saving my money and I'm pretty sure I'll have enough by the time you go back to Arizona. Don't forget that I want to buy your board."

He was shrewd and I was naive. He knew exactly how to make me feel anxious. He fanned my desire for that board until I just had to have it. When he left, I handed him $60 (13 of them in change) and he handed me a battered hulk with a splintered nose, dings in the rails, and a skeg that wobbled like a loose tooth. It was a worthless piece of junk, but I didn't know that at the time. I was happy learning to surf on it, and that's all that really matters.

"We lost you last year because of that accident, and it looks like we're going to lose you this year because of surfing. Why do you run around with that grubby-looking bunch of long-haired bums?"

The coach wasn't pleased. He gave me all sorts of reasons for giving up surfing and concentrating on running. Paddling would hurt my knees. I'd get bumps on my feet that would blister in my shoes. The cold water would make my legs cramp up. Above all, surfers were lazy and irresponsible. Runners were hard-working and disciplined. It should be obvious where I belonged.

The other runners weren't pleased, either. If I spent time surfing, I was letting the team down. They complained in good humor, but I could tell they really meant it. When they met me in the hallways, they would greet me with cries of "Surfer!" From the tone of their voices, they might as well have been saying "Traitor!"

I couldn't understand what the fuss was all about, because I was not a good runner. As a schoolboy in England, and then Canada, I had played soccer. In California, running was the only sport I could enjoy. I was too light for football, too short for basketball and uninterested in baseball.

When playing soccer, I had loved the continuous ebb and flow of the game. I had loved getting carried away by the action and yet feeling that everything I did counted. In running, I got that same feeling of personal importance, but I could never get really caught up in racing. In fact, racing made me feel like a failure.

Race days were one long agony of anticipation. Walking up to the starting line was a real ordeal. And each race followed the same dismal pattern.

"Those guys are so much bigger and stronger than I am. I wonder if I even have a chance. It'll take three of my strides to make two of theirs.

"The gun! I've got to stay with them. If I fall behind, I'll never be able to catch up."

Somehow or other, I had picked up the idea that running was a matter of enduring pain, and the best and fastest runners were simply braver than the rest of us. As I watched them smoothly pull away from me, in spite of my desperate efforts, in spite of my aching legs and burning lungs, I felt that I was being exposed as a failure. They had it and I didn't.

"You've got to have guts!" screamed the coach. "Get that man! Catch him! All you need is guts!"

The notice above the bulletin board said, "When the going gets tough, the tough get going." It was always the first thing I saw when I hobbled back into the locker room. Each time, it was an accusation. "You just don't have what it takes. You're not tough enough."

At the same time, I thought I was doing my best, but I couldn't be sure. When I ran the 440 intervals in training, I would wait for the pain to start and then try to master it. It was like trying to run in waist deep treacle. It was hopeless. But I had been led to believe that all I needed was inner toughness. I was convinced that everyone who ran faster was going through the same pain but had resources of strength and courage that I lacked.

"If I can't even face the challenge of a race," I thought, "what's going to happen when I'm out of school and into the world? If I can't cope here, what's going to happen to me out there?"

Sam liked me because I had an English accent and I wasn't as good on a surfboard as he was. I liked Sam because he had a Chevy Impala with white tuck-and-roll upholstery and surfboard racks. He had an olive complexion, jet black hair, a hooked nose and an infectious smile. On weekends, we would drive up and down the coast, searching for surf. One Friday night, we drove down to San Diego to see a movie called "Search for Surf."

There was a screen set up in front of the stage. Someone was adjusting a projector near the back of the hall. In the din of shuffling feet and the hardwood scrape of folding chairs, we moved as close to the front as we could. Bottle caps were spinning through the air. There was plenty of long blond hair. The girls looked beautifully tanned and totally inaccessible.

The lights dimmed. Hearty cheering and stamping of feet. On the screen, nothing but featureless blurred green. Then silence. More silence. Then fidgeting and mumbling. Was something wrong with the projector?

Then suddenly there was life. The hall exploded with a raucous, gutty, rock-and-roll instrumental. The screen came into sharp focus and the green blur become a massive wall of water, moving in slow motion like the flank of a huge beast in labor.

And there was a man riding it. He dropped in from the top of the screen, crouched low over his board, driving down and across that heaving green. Two, three, four times his height he dropped down into that wave. He desperately trimmed his board for speed, but an avalanche of white water buried him before he could reach the shoulder.

Pandemonium broke loose. As one body, we jumped on our chairs, roaring and screaming in ecstatic disbelief. I felt swallowed up in powerful feelings, sucked into an unknown that was vaguely threatening. I had a lump in my throat and tears in my eyes, and I felt marvellously alive. How was it humanly possible to dare? How was it possible to survive those giant waves?

The incredible kept unfolding on the screen. Wave after wave towered ominously over a dwarf crouched on a sliver of a surfboard.

"You judge the size of those waves," said the narrator. "Those boards are 11 and 12 feet long. When you're after elephants, you need an elephant gun. When you're after big waves, you need a big gun too, and you'd better be made of iron."

The close-ups were absolutely hair-raising. You could see how the offshore wind ripped the sleeting spray off the crest of the wave. You could see how furiously the men had to paddle to get into the waves. You could see the boards lurch as the waves picked them up. You could see them carving savage trails as they fought to beat the thunderous collapse. You could see mere humans inserting them-selves into significance. You could see life grabbing them in the guts and squeezing the moment into the wine of terror.

2 What Are You Made Of ?

"All the statistics and studies show the same thing," said the counsellor. "The more education you have, the more money you can expect to make over a lifetime of earning. If your grades are good enough, you should definitely go on to college. If they aren't, then work on them."

The fall after graduation from high school, I found myself caught up in the confusion of college registration. Working out a schedule of classes turned into a nightmare, even though signing up for the cross-country team had earned me "athletic priority" and an early registration time. I waited in one wrong line after another. I ran around from department to department, trying to get into classes that didn't conflict with each other. I needed Psychology 1, and I couldn't find out where to sign up for it.

"Where's psychiatry?" I blurted out. "All I need is psychiatry to get my program together."

The man at the information desk appraised me with his mild eyes. A sweaty, harassed freshman clutching a wad of IBM cards and caught up in a panic of urgency. I could read it in his face, "I wonder how long this character is going to last."

"If you want psychiatry," he said with irritating deliberation. "We have a little room downstairs and consultation will be $25 an hour. But if you want to get a psychology class, the line is over there by the door."

It was not a promising beginning.

And things didn't get any better. College was supposed to be preparation for entering the mainstream of adult life. It was supposed to be some sort of a passport to the good life. You went to classes, you studied, you took exams, you earned a degree. Then you got a job, you got married, you bought a house in the suburbs with a two-car garage and you had a couple of kids. Once you had done all that, you were a success. You could invite your friends over and display your success to them.

That kind of success didn't interest me. Although I went to classes regularly, I couldn't get over the feeling that I was just marking time.

Nothing I had seen of the adult success game was attractive. It has been called a rat-race, and for good reason, it seemed to me. But it was all that was offered. I knew of no other game to play. One part of me rejected it totally as meaningless and absurd. Another part of me worried that I wouldn't be able to make the grade. "This is what life is all about," it said, "so stop your complaining and get down to work."

It's not easy to get to work when you don't believe in what you are doing. The struggle to make it in the modern world looked demanding enough. Failure was a real and frightening possibility. But failure seemed a certainty for anyone whose heart wasn't in the struggle. Each day seemed to bring me closer not to success and security, but to an inevitable showdown with my inadequacy.

That's why cross-country and track became so important for me. I hoped that racing would teach me to tap those inner resources of will and courage, and with that power I would be able to do anything.

My approach to track and cross-country was much the same in college as it had been in high school. Each workout and each race brought me face to face with that nagging question, "Are you tough enough?"

I believed that if I could force myself to do everything the coach told me to, if I could throw myself completely into the running, then somehow, sometime, I would grow tough and confident—not only for racing, but for the larger challenges of life.

In high school, the cross-country workouts had been simplicity itself—twice around the course as fast as we could run. College workouts were much more involved, and much more demanding. We ran long intervals round an enormous field. We did repeat hills on a road leading up to the parking lots. Occasionally, we went to the mountains to run the rough trails. The coach ran with us.

"Let's push these uphill sections! Drive! Drive! I want to see you pick it up coming off the top. I don't care how your legs feel. Just grit your teeth and push. We're going to win the conference title again this year, and we're going to do it with our strength on hills."

He was an amazing man. He shamed us into giving our best. If he could run along with us, shouting and cussing us, then the least we could do was to try to stay up with him. I can still remember that fierce quality in his voice, harsh, strident, decisive. It convinced me that he was really into something, that he himself had gone through the initiation of pain and was now as strong as tempered steel. The power of his personality was a bright light. If I could only stick with it, running under him would really make me grow.

"Now I want you guys to be tough," the coach said. "For each one of you, this has to be the best race of your life. We can win the title if everyone comes through. And I mean everyone." His eyes caught mine. "The fifth man might be the deciding factor. Don't let your teammates down."

We were at the Mt. Sac Invitational. The sun was bright. Hot, gusty winds picked up the dust and whirled it into our faces. I looked around the track and over at the field with the limed starting line. The runners were a swirl of bright colors. I loosened up a little and joined in the milling flow of the warm up. There were red sweats and blue and yellow and green. Everyone looked lean and hungry, businesslike, professional, competent. And as I took off my sweats, it occurred to me that I must look just as much a real runner as everyone else there. That was exciting.

Ernie Portee, our top runner, came up to me as we moved to the starting line. "I think we can do it. Just give it all you've got. I know I can count on you."

That friendly gesture made me feel wonderful. Suddenly, I wasn't fighting pre-race panic so much. I knew that he was going to push himself to his limit, and I was determined to do the same. There was a chance that I would be fifth man on the team. If I didn't finish well, I would be letting him down.

I knelt behind the line, double-knotting my laces. My mouth was dry. The skin on my back was prickling under the nylon singlet. "I'm really going to break through in this race," I promised myself. "I'm going to push every step. When I cross that finish line, I'm going to be completely spent."

The start of the race was brutal. We surged across a dusty field at a blistering pace, and then thundered over a wooden bridge. Approaching the bridge, we had to funnel down. No one wanted to lose position, so there was plenty of free elbowing. Past the bridge, we came to the first hill, and that's where my resolution was first tested.

Somehow, I had been carried along by the momentum of the start, and I was up with the fourth man on the team. "I'm going to stay with him," I told myself. "If I have to fight it every step of the way, I'm going to stay with him."

But a gap opened up, and it grew steadily wider. It was five, and then 10, and then 15 yards.

"You've got to get in contact again. You can do it. Forget the pain. You can stand it for one more step, and then another one after that, and then all the steps to the finish line. This is it. This is where you discover what you are really made of."

I fixed my eyes on the small of his back and summoned all my will power to pull myself towards it. I gained a couple of yards and then I lost it. No matter how hard I tried, I couldn't close that gap. Finally, I lost sight of him, but I kept forcing myself at every step, trying to stay with the runners close by me.

After what seemed an endless struggle, the trail approached the track. The end was in sight.

"Just one lap!" shouted the coach as I went by him. 'Don't be a quitter! Don't let up! Catch that man in front of you!"

He had about 30 yards on me, and I couldn't gain on him. My legs felt like logs. I could barely lift my knees. But on the final turn, he slowed to a walk. Hope gave me a sudden surge of energy, and I managed a shambling sprint to the finish line.

As I staggered around the infield, fighting the dry heaves, I was blaming myself for failure. Why had I let that gap open up in the first place? If I had really confronted the pain right at the beginning, I could have conquered it and stayed up with that fourth man. How much had I been kidding myself about the effort? If I had really been pushing myself to my limit, where had I found the energy for a kick?

Ernie was walking along beside me. "How did you do?" I asked him. "How did we do?"

"I came in third and the first count shows that we won, by one point. When you beat that guy on the last turn, you sewed it up for us. That was a great effort."

I knew he was just trying to make me feel good, but I appreciated it anyway. I knew that his effort had been far greater than anything I was capable of. It was by far my best race, but it sank me even deeper into self-doubt.

3 On the Treadmill of Challenge

The exhaust pipes glowed in the dark. The wings rippled in the bumpy air. The engines droned on. I stared vacantly out the window. My mind, like the airliner, was poised midway between where I had been and where I was going.

Behind me was California, students cramming for finals, unsuspecting parents, and desperate confusion. Beneath me, in the cargo section of the plane, was my surfboard and a suitcase full of clothes. Ahead in the darkness lay the Hawaiian Islands, giant surf and a pressing question, "Do you have what it takes?"

I thought back to my interview with the Dean of Students. "I think your decision is foolish," he said. "I'm sure you're going to regret it. Why don't you think about it until finals are over and then come back and discuss it?"

"If I stay for finals, I'm admitting that I think all this stuff is important." I said. "If I stay for finals, I'll end up staying forever. I feel totally inadequate and I've got to strike out on my own."

"But why Hawaii? What will you find there that you don't have here? We take our problems around with us, you know. A change of place is not going to bring about a change of heart."

"In the first place," I said, "Hawaii is 2500 miles of Pacific Ocean from here. When I'm in Hawaii, I'll be on my own, and I won't be able to hitchhike home when I get hungry. I simply can't cope right now. I don't have what it takes. Being on my own will force me to cope, and when I've gained confidence and self-respect, I'll be able to come back and finish my education."

"But if you just buckle down and work on your finals right now, you can prove to yourself that you *can* cope. You can prove it without going off half-cocked to a testing ground 2500 miles across the ocean. Why postpone the showdown? Why make a special arena for yourself? Don't be a quitter. You have a week till finals start. In that time you can show yourself that you *do* have what it takes."

"I've already made my plane reservation," I said. "I'm going to keep it. Please approve my withdrawal form. I'm not going to change my mind."

"No. If you want to drop out now, you'll have to take the consequences of Fs in all your courses. I'm sorry, but that's the way it has to be. I won't sign that card."

And as I thought back over that conversation, I was still surprised at my reaction. Suddenly I had felt the power of real decision.

"If that's what it's going to cost me, I'll pay it. You have your responsibility and I have mine. My responsibility is to work this problem out in the way I see fit. Thank you for your time. Shall I throw these cards away, or leave them with the secretary?"

"No. Wait. Give them to me," he said. "I'll sign them, and I wish you luck in your quest. I still think you're making a mistake, but I admire your pluck anyway."

Pluck he had called it. I wondered how plucky he would think me if he knew how scared I was right now. I didn't know whether I was taking steps to suicide or to life.

I vividly remembered the incredible scenes of big surf from that movie. That, to me, was the ultimate challenge. If I could handle the terror of big surf, I would be able to handle anything. If I could not, then drowning was a clean and a sure way to die.

"Look at this!" said Larry. "We're the stars of the show and we can't even find a parking space."

The road that rims the bay was packed with cars and tour buses. There were at least eight telephoto barrels trained on the handful of surfers off the north point, and other cameramen were setting up their equipment. We squeezed into an opening and hurriedly pulled the boards off the racks. As we weaved through the crowd with our boards, Larry was clowning irrepressibly. I didn't feel in the mood. I was torn between fear of the waves and longing for them.

"We're going to have to wait for a lull before we can get out through the shorebreak. Let's just relax and put some more wax on the boards. Your new board really needs it."

I put mine down in the sand. It had cost me all but $20 of my survival savings, but it was worth every penny. Long and slender, with a pointed nose, a good belly and a tapering tail, it was the right kind of gun for hunting elephants. I rubbed the wax in vigorously, losing myself in the energy of the motion.

"Any time now," said Larry.

He picked up his board and ran down the steep beach. Throwing the board lightly on the flow of the backwash, he pushed out with a smooth swing and paddled hard through the inshore turbu-

lence. I followed him. We settled down for the long paddle out to
the point.

"How do you feel?"

"Scared." I couldn't put flippancy in my voice.

"Don't think about it. Just do it."

Don't think about it. Just do it. That might be good advice for
many things beside riding big waves. I noticed the spectators along
the black rocks, pointing. The horizon was convulsing. A big set was
on the way.

We picked up the rhythm. Larry was about 20 yards in front of
me. About 50 yards beyond him, I could see the handful of surfers
jockeying for position. Beyond the group, I could see the first wave
of the set starting to climb as it moved over the deep reefs.

As they all paddled over it, I realized how enormous the wave
was. Suddenly, I felt a dreamy detachment. I couldn't believe that
I was really out at Waimea Bay, facing my first big wave.

"It's mine!" I yelled to Larry, leaning back on the tailblock and
pulling the nose around. With a glance back over my shoulder, I began an accelerating paddle rhythm. The board was sucked back up
the wave. It seemed to get cranked up higher with every stroke I
took. At the top, I could feel the wind trying to get under the belly
of the board. The last few strokes were a wild windmill flurry. Then
the board lurched down. I was up, crouched against the wind and
the bumpy waveface.

The board was fast, stable and responsive. Although the ride
was just an elevator drop and a touch-and-go drive to beat the white-
water, it seemed to take an eternity.

If you've ever had a close brush with death, a near head-on col-
lision or a violent spinout on a wet road, you know the feeling that
shot through my body. It was a pure adrenalin flash. Pure and hard
and heavy. As I pulled out over the shoulder of the wave, I balanced
for a moment in ecstasy. Then my knees buckled and I toppled into
the warm water, laughing uproariously. It was an instant addiction.
Still laughing, I paddled back to the lineup.

I spent three winters in the Islands, living a life that must have
been the dream of thousands of surfers. After the first six months, I
rarely worked. I lived out on the North Shore, the surfer's Mecca,
where each winter brought the North Pacific storms, the giant surf,
the pilgrimage of devotees and armies of surf photographers with
telephoto cannons. When I got up in the morning, I could walk out

into the garden and watch the frosty peaks of Sunset Beach steaming in.

The center of my life was the gutty excitement of riding big waves; I loved putting myself in situations where I couldn't think about what I was doing, where there was no time for anything but decisive action. I always sought out the challenge of the biggest, the steepest, the fastest, the most powerful waves. The love affair with danger seemed to have no end.

But it wore thin. The adrenalin kick got diluted. I hungered for bigger challenges. So I set out on what was to have been a round the world odyssey by stowing away on a ship to Australia. When I got caught in Sydney and was sent back to the Islands, I tried escalating the challenge by taking heavy doses of LSD before paddling out into massive surf. I narrowly escaped with my life on two occasions.

After the last of these, my nerve failed me. I could not push the stakes any higher. I wrote my parents for help in finishing my college degree. There was never any question about it. They welcomed my return without even a hint of recrimination.

4 Hawaiian Print Tennies.

"Jackson," he said. "I want to talk to you. Sit down for a minute."

I panicked. He was going to be handing back our first test today, and I was sure I had done miserably. He pushed his tray aside. Placing my books on the table, I sat down across from him. I tried to read his eyes through his dark glasses. What could this brilliant man have to say to me? Was he going to hint diplomatically that I wasn't up to his intellectual standards? Was he going to suggest that I withdraw from his class?

"I'm going to do you a favor, Jackson. You can see your paper an hour before class." He handed it to me. I didn't want to look at the grade, but I was obviously supposed to. *Beowulf: the Image of the Hero.* Grade: A. I felt a shock of pleasant surprise.

"I know from the way you write that you've been around," he said. "Tell me about yourself. How did you get that kind of insight?"

I read where he had put check marks in the margin.

"In the time of Beowulf, there was space enough for naked, blunt, superb heroism. Grendel, the monster Beowulf challenges and slays, symbolizes the endless pressure of immediate danger, the absolute hostility of the environment. We have horrors as great and inscrutable as Grendel. We live in constant fear of atomic holocaust. But we can't go out to slay our monsters. The modern world is far too complex for that."

I pointed the section out to him. "This is rather evasive," I said. "I have lived in fear for many years, but not because of the threat of atomic orgy. It's more a fear of life itself, of my incapacity to meet its demands. I've just returned from Hawaii, where I tried to come to terms with fear by riding big surf."

"I thought you were a surfer," he said. "You dress in a very distinctive way."

I turned red. All I was wearing was a torn T-shirt and a ragged pair of Bermuda trunks. I was acutely aware of the cold floor under my bare feet. I escaped into the paper again.

"Each threat was a showdown with the possibility of defeat," I had written. "Beowulf and his warriors shored up their sense of identity by boasting and bragging in the safety of the Mead Hall. But each knew that he had only the strength of his arm and the sharpness of his sword to rely on.

"Each of them had to seek out new challenges, new monsters, in order to uphold his self-respect and reputation. But there is an intolerable boredom and an agony of compulsion in the need constantly to throw down the gauntlet to future challenges. To live by facing danger is to take on a burden that becomes heavier at each step. When you have to meet challenges to define your worth, you have no time for anything outside the arena of challenge, no time for exploring any other possibilities of life."

I pointed out that section to him. "That's why I'm here now, and not still on the North Shore, where my Grendel is, in the big surf."

"Look, Jackson," he said decisively. "A guy like you doesn't have any business wasting his time. I want you to be my assistant. The English department wants me to use grad students, but you have more on the ball than they do. I'll be able to get you on. There's one condition, though."

He paused reflectively. "What's it going to be?" I thought.

"You have to clean yourself up. I can't be associated with a seedy bum like you. Get a shave, get a haircut, get some nice clothes. I'll meet you here at 10 tomorrow. I've got some papers for you to correct."

When I met him next day, I was shaved and shorn. I had blown all my money on a sportscoat, shirt, tie and slacks. I even had shoes and socks on. I couldn't go all the way, though. I had to have at least a toehold in chaos. Instead of dress shoes, I wore a pair of Hawaiian print tennies.

My path was blocked, but I was too intrigued to be irritated. Pouring out of the classroom, through the bushes and onto the lawn was a stream of students. Old and young, hip and square, surf nymphs and sorority girls—all of them shining with blissful radiance. My first thought was that they were all on acid.

A girl cut in front of me. Yellow shift, golden hair, warmly tanned shoulders. As if in a dream, she reached out to touch a tree trunk. Her fingertips played gently on the rough bark. I was close enough to hear the hushed wonder in her voice.

"It's really here. I'm really alive!"

My eyes lingered on her smooth back. Then the movement

around us drew them away. Beside me stood a bearded man, entranced. Sunlight glinted off his gold-trimmed glasses. His hands, held loosely at his sides, were slowly opening. His fingers spread slowly, with a life of their own.

A slight, silver-haired lady stopped under an arch. She stooped to put her books on the pathway and then slowly straightened. Like a cat easing its way out of sleep, she stretched her arms out. She arched her back and let the sun play on her eyelids and on her blissful smile.

The golden girl had clear blue eyes. She touched me with them as she had touched the tree with her fingertips. I felt an immediate flush. Something surged across the space between us like a spark jumping a gap: "I'm really here! You're really here! How wonderful!"

Too shy to talk to her, I watched the teacher through the door-way as he gathered his books. He was short and dark, solidly and compactly built. With his bristling moustache, he looked like a fierce zen master—an intense, decisive man who would brook no nonsense.

As I watched him cross the courtyard, I sensed that he knew ex-actly where he was and why. He knew exactly what he was doing, and exactly where he was going. The very rhythm of his walk spoke of a deep calmness within.

Next semester, when I planned my class schedule, I did some jug-gling so that I could include his class on Indian philosophy. During that semester, there were two magical lectures, but I experienced on-ly a mild degree of ecstasy. I wanted more. I wanted to be able to lose myself in blissful consciousness, to enter samadhi, that ecstatic cosmic consciousness I had been reading so much about. I guess I was too greedy, or perhaps too hung up on intellectual understanding.

I read and reread the assignments. I always had plenty of paper on hand for notes. Throughout each lecture, I listened eagerly for gems of oriental wisdom. Most of the time, my head was bent over the desk as my pencil scratched feverishly across the page.

And most of the time, I would end up scratching my head over those notes. In my other courses, grasping the ideas was as easy as picking up a rock. In this course, the ideas were like slippery bars of soap. I'd lose them in the very effort of grasping them.

The most slippery soap was yoga. For the midterm, we had to connect the following two verses from the Bhagavad Gita according to the Indian vision of right action:

On action alone be thy interest,
Never on its fruits;

> *Let not the fruits of action be thy motive,*
> *Nor be thy attachment to inaction.*

> *Holding pleasure and pain alike,*
> *Gain and loss, victory and defeat,*
> *Then gird thyself for battle:*
> *Thus thou shalt not get evil.*

During the lectures, I had strained my brain to understand those verses. I had put tremendous effort into listening for a new idea or a well-turned phrase that would make everything come clear. I had covered many pages with my scribbling.

When I worked on that question, I *really* worked, or so I thought. We were limited to three pages of double-spaced typing. It's incredible how difficult ideas can be when they have to be expressed with both clarity and brevity. Then those bars of soap take on a life of their own.

I wrote and revised again and again. Finally, I had what I thought was a real gem—three tightly-written pages that focussed my understanding. Not a word was wasted. Even the syllables had been adjusted for rhythm and smooth reading. I counted my pages of revisions when I was finished. It had taken me 106 to produce those three.

For all that work, the grade was B. Not a B+ or an A-, but a straight B! I went up to his office in dismay. Where had I gone wrong?

"I know exactly how you wrote this paper, " he told me. "You went home and you slaved over those notes I see you busily jotting down. The writing is smooth and competent, but it doesn't say anything. You made a major effort of sticking sentences and phrases together and sanding down the rough edges. I can recognize my own lectures, you know."

What could I say? He was absolutely right. But it had never occurred to me that I should try to face the question alone, without the help of my notes.

"You could have been using those notes all along to generate the energy of exploration," he said. "Instead, you have been wasting time playing with them, never venturing out beyond them."

What can you do when you're busted like that? It's useless to pretend that the truth isn't there. I asked him how to go about flexing my intelligence independently.

"I can't give you a special way," he said. "You have to discover that for yourself. My suggestion is for you to work with those two verses. There's enough in those verses for a lifetime."

5   Blood on the Floor

The spring semester was over. The studying was over, and the lectures and examinations. A friend and I were driving out to school to clear out our P.E. lockers.

"This is going to be a great summer," he was saying. "There's a south swell building right now. It's a good beginning."

"I'm glad it's all over for a few months," I said. "The boss has me scheduled for the jeep next Monday. When do you start?"

"What the..."

I caught a glimpse of his knuckles on the steering wheel. I sensed something flying at us. Then I went into a slow motion dream. Crashes echoed into each other.

As my head floated back from the windshield, I noticed the shatter lines, sparkling, still spreading outwards. I noticed the color of the car ploughed head-on into the hood. Red. I thought, "Fire! Get out!"

Stumbling onto the shoulder of the road, I saw red blood streaming down my shirt. My mouth felt funny. I explored with my tongue. No more front teeth, just blubbery gums. I gingerly felt my lower lip It had somehow been hooked over the lower teeth. I could feel one of them protruding through it.

The emergency room was a blur of harsh lights, shiny chrome, and white sheets. The stranger who had given me a ride turned and ran. I wandered dazedly around, looking for help.

An orderly grabbed my shoulder from behind, spun me around into the hatred of his eyes. "Watch what you're doing," he screamed. "I don't want this blood all over my floor."

His voice was bitchy. Womanish. I hated his guts.

It was a brutal nightmare. I had been looking forward to another summer of life-guarding, another long and loose rest from the pressures of school. When the damage had been assessed, that summer dream was obviously out of the question. My jaw had been broken, some upper and lower front teeth had snapped off at the gum line and my right knee was so severely battered by something under the dashboard I could barely walk on it.

When I got out of the hospital, I felt like a cripple. With my jaws wired together, I couldn't do anything active because I couldn't suck in enough air through the gap in my front teeth. Even when the wires were taken out, I was still crippled. My knee wouldn't support more than a few blocks of easy walking.

Forced suddenly into inactivity, I quickly lost my physical condition. And I didn't like it one bit.

"Now I understand why the drug industry makes so much money," I told my friends. "If all those people who live by elevators and automobiles feel the way I do now, it's no wonder they spend billions each year on aspirins, pep pills and tranquilizers."

I began to have headaches. I sank into chronic fatigue, dullness and lethargy. One day, my lifeguarding buddy from the Islands came by to try getting me out of the doldrums.

"The boss says that if you think you can handle it you can work the last few weeks of summer. You're not going to pick up many girls with those broken teeth of yours, but at least you can start getting in shape again."

"You're kidding," I said. "I thought I had been written off till next year. Can I start tomorrow?"

I was down at the beach next morning, ready to get up in a tower.

"Now there's one thing I want to be sure about," said the boss. "Is this accident going to cut down your abilities in any way? Greg tells me you have a bad knee. Can you jump down from a tower without hurting it? Will you be able to make a fast run on a rescue?"

I climbed up in a tower and managed to get down passably well by swinging from the ladder instead of jumping straight onto the sand. I sprinted to the water's edge and managed to hide the knee pain as I walked back.

"OK," he said. "Put your trunks on and go to tower three. People are already beginning to arrive."

I got up in the tower, hoping that I would be up to anything I had to handle. As it turned out, the excitement of rescues always blotted out the knee pain. However, "getting in shape again" was no easy matter.

"More knee problems?" Greg asked as I came limping back to the headquarters. "Why do you keep at it when you just end up hurting yourself?"

"It may hurt now, but I'm hoping to push through it. If I give in, I'm afraid I might start a long slide into the miserable shape of the average guy on the street."

By the time the fall semester came around, I had made little progress with the knee. I'd go out onto the track, always hoping for a miracle, but never able to run more than one lap. Running made the knee feel as if there were tight hot wires inside the joint itself, binding it up. There was no pushing through. Continued running made the pain unbearably intense.

On the other hand, I could swim freestyle without difficulty. If the knee felt at all sensitive, I just let the legs trail in the water. By the time I had worked up to a daily 1000 yards, I was feeling in reasonably comfortable condition. I vowed I would never let myself slide into that hell of poor condition again.

"It seems like you take a few seconds off your 1000 time every week," said the pool guard. "You must be working really hard on that."

"Thanks," I said, surprised that anyone had noticed. "I like to be in shape. I had a bad accident at the beginning of last summer. I couldn't do anything for months, and I couldn't believe how low it made me feel. There's one thing that worries me now, though. I don't know what I'll do without a pool. My knee is so weak that swimming is my only exercise."

"Have you thought about having an operation? Maybe they could just go into there and straighten things out."

I had thought about an operation, but had held back. The idea of having a surgeon's scalpel cutting into my knee made me nauseous. Besides, when I tried running, I sometimes found that I could go as far as two laps before the knee started hurting.

The orthopedic surgeon I saw wasn't impressed at these small signs of improvement. He looked closely at the x-rays. His frown made me very uncomfortable.

"The knee's stress tolerance will of course vary, but with this condition you're going to have to resign yourself to an overall pattern of deterioration. I can understand your reluctance to have an operation. You can always give me a call when it gets really bad. But I don't see why you want to postpone it. Why suffer needlessly?"

The track coach wasn't much impressed by the orthopedist's diagnosis.

"I've heard stories about that guy. He's a scalpel-happy butcher. Talk to the new trainer before you decide. If you do go for an operation, stay away from the butcher."

The trainer was young and dynamic. After manipulating my knee for a while to find out which movements caused pain, he showed me some exercises to correct the problem.

"There's nothing we can do about the joint itself, but we can do plenty with the supporting muscles, especially the quadriceps. You can work on these exercises, and you can also do some repeat runs up the stairs. If the stair runs are too difficult to start with, try wading back and forth across the shallow end of the pool with high knee lift."

By following his advice, I was able to improve the knee, but not to overcome the problem entirely. Perhaps I was too impatient, and put too much pressure on it too soon. Whatever the reason, I still had to take occasional layoffs and return to swimming laps in the pool.

6 A Warm Pool of Blue

It was still totally dark outside. It was raining heavily. Steam rose off the water and drifted up into the mist. In the floodlights, the pool looked like a heavenly blue refuge. One by one, we dashed through the cold and dived into the warm of that clean, well-lighted place.

The coach walked out onto the deck. He was wearing a hooded parka, heavy boots, thick mittens and a scarf wound up to his eyes. He huddled with his stopwatches under a broken-ribbed umbrella. His voice was flat and muffled through the scarf.

"OK, let's loosen up! Swim 400, kick 200—easy."

Easy and relaxed. I relished the lazy feel of my recovering arm arcing through the air, the crisp splash of my hand plunging into the water, the fluid pull/push resistance on the power arm, the loose heaviness of the flutter kick.

After the 400, I grabbed a kickboard off the deck. Curving my forearms around the edges and resting my chin on the back, I settled into the 200 kick. I relished the feel and sound of the big raindrops splattering into my wet hair and splashing into the water by my ears. I relished the coach's shouts echoing into the steady beat of the kicking, and the warm ache that spread into my shoulders and thighs.

The workouts usually lasted from 1½ to two hours. By the time we pulled ourselves out of the pool and ran inside for hot showers, the dawn would be breaking.

It was demanding, exhausting work, but I loved it anyway. Afterwards, on the long walk up campus to the library, I would feel tired, but also fresh, clean and alive. When one of the swimmers asked me why I always worked so hard ("As a grad student, you're not even eligible to compete"), I pointed to the students hunched over the cafeteria tables, waking themselves up with cigarettes and coffee.

"I don't want to feel like those poor bastards. It's happened to me once, and I don't want it to happen again."

But there was more to it than that—much more. Whenever I pushed through the heavy doors of Wheeler Hall, I lost those feelings of purity and certainty. The very atmosphere of the place transformed the relaxed swimmer into an uptight academic.

I woke up with a start. Julia was standing by my side, her hand on my shoulder.

"Are you feeling all right?" she said.

She was trying—and failing—not to look overly concerned. We both knew it.

"This is the fourth night in a row you've fallen asleep over your books. Are you just tired, or are you worried about something? Do you want to talk about it?"

I didn't want to talk about it. I didn't want to admit it to myself. I didn't want to admit it to her. I didn't want to face it.

"Nothing's wrong," I said. "I need more sleep. That's all."

"You do need more sleep. But there's something else, too. What happened to all the enthusiasm you had when you got your fellowship after our wedding? What happened to all your interest? You're putting more energy into swimming than studying. I don't think you realize what it's doing to you. Why don't you admit it was a mistake to come here? Why don't you do something else? Drop out and get a job. Find out what you're interested in. I don't care whether you teach in a university or drive a bus.   All that matters is that you do what you really want to do.

I didn't want to talk about it. I was too tired. I couldn't think clearly.

"I don't want to drop out. What would I do then? I'd lose my fellowship. How much money do we have in the bank? Not even $20. We'd be in deep trouble."

"No we wouldn't. You'd just go out and get a job like everyone else does. You'd work eight hours a day, you'd make good money, and you'd be able to come home at night and relax. You wouldn't have to worry any more about papers and exams, and we wouldn't have to live like paupers any more.

"I don't know how you can stand the pressure. If you really want that Ph.D., then do what you're supposed to do. Really put your heart into it. Stop escaping into diversions like swimming."

I focused my eyes on the words I had fallen asleep over. There was no life in them. I couldn't feel them the way I could feel cold concrete, sleeting rain and aching muscles. The university was to the big world outside what the lighted pool was to the early morning darkness. It was a place of security, a refuge I didn't want to leave. Even though it was turning into a nightmare, it was at least a familiar nightmare, less frightening than the unknown.

7 A Different Kind of LSD

I had just finished my toughest running workout in several years —five 440s in about 70 seconds each, with an easy 440 walk recovery. I was walking back up to the gym with a friend.

"I'm jealous," he said. "You've hardly been doing any running at all and yet you don't even look tired. I'm completely wiped out."

"Don't forget, that I've been swimming many thousands of yards a day for the past several months. At least I have basic condition; that makes it much easier on me. I'm wondering how much longer I'll be able to keep this up, though. My right knee has been bad since I smashed it up in a head-on car crash several years ago. I thought it might have healed up with all that swimming, but I'm feeling those old twinges again after today's run."

I was walking very carefully, trying to avoid the painful leg actions. My friend was suddenly thoughtful.

"Hey!" he said. "I know what I meant to suggest today! I've just read two great running books that have a whole new approach. We should be going slow and long instead of running these hard intervals. I brought them along to lend you. I bet they'll help you handle your knee problems."

I went by his locker after showering and dressing. He was stuffing his running shoes into his knapsack.

"They're in the back, under the towel," he said as he shook the knapsack down. "The ideas sound pretty radical, but they make sense. I want the books back by next week. I know some other guys who might be interested."

"Thanks," I said. "I'll read them right away."

I looked them over as I walked on up to the library: *The Conditioning of Distance Runners*, by Tom Osler, and *LSD: The Humane Way to Train*, by Joe Henderson. When I sat down at my study carrel, I pushed my English books aside and read the running books from cover to cover.

Those two slim books were worth more to me than stacks of academic work. If what they said was true, if my problems could be as easily overcome as they suggested, it could make all the difference in the world. I could use running as a pleasant way to keep in good condition. I would never again have to worry about sinking into the hell of poor health.

Osler said, *"Injury and illness are the result of overtaxing one's energy reserves and are, in almost all cases, not the result of accident.* A properly conditioned runner, whose body can handle even more than the daily training load, is virtually 'injury and sickness proof.' You may ask, 'Is not stepping on a stone and twisting one's ankle an accident?' I'd answer, emphatically, 'No!'

"A fresh runner is: (a) alert and quick to avoid trouble; (b) in possession of quick reflexes to respond to a possible sprain; (c) sufficiently healthy to recover quickly from minor sprains and strains. On the other hand, a tired runner is: (a) sluggish and non-observant of possible trouble; (b) dull and unable to react in time to avoid a sprain; (c) run-down generally and unable to recover from minor problems which in turn may develop into serious injuries."

I knew that my knee injury might be too severe to be solved by simply staying fresh. I also knew that the combination of swimming and running I was doing at the time was a major physical load. Perhaps the knee would hold up if I cut down on the load by running at a slow pace, as Osler recommended.

The running biographies in Joe Henderson's book gave me more hope. Besides his own running experiences, Joe described those of Jeff Kroot, Tom Osler, Bob Deines, Ed Winrow and Amby Burfoot. They had all discovered the same thing—slow training eliminates injuries and, unbelievable as it may sound, leads to fast racing.

Here's how Henderson explained it:

"Speed, the speed needed to race adequately at distances longer than a mile, anyway, is quickly sharpened down to the limits of our ingrained abilities. After reaching that point, additional speed training is of dubious value. And worse, it hurts. It hurries the rush of fatigue-producing lactic acid through the muscles. And it raises the risk of stress injuries—pulled muscles, strained tendons, fatigue fractures and the like—until the user hovers at the danger line.

"I'm oversimplifying the situation, but it's basically true that fast running hurts, and the faster one goes the more it's likely to hurt. Hurting isn't much fun under any circumstances."

Joe made it clear that the approach he was advocating was controversial:

"Rich Delgado, who blasts through his 140 miles a week seldom seeing the slow side of 6:00 a mile, takes friendly offense at my pro-

moting the idea of slowness. He claims he is going to write a counter-
ing article called 'POT—Plenty of Tempo.'

In Rich's terms, and he undoubtedly represents the majority,
the 'best' system is one which produces the fastest racing times and
the highest placings most quickly."

"Slow down and live!" Henderson and Osler seemed to be saying.
With my many years of hard workouts in high school and college, I
found this advice radically new—and radically appealing. If my right
knee had been able, I'm sure it would have been urging, "Do it! Do
it!"

It held up very well with the new way of running. Not even a
murmur of protest. As long as I stayed at a gentle, relaxed pace, the
knee was quiet and contented. When occasionally I pushed into the
danger zone, the push was so easy and tentative that I could hear the
whispered warnings in time to back down. In the middle of a flat-out
440, all I could hear was pounding feet and heavy breathing. Under
those circumstances, I was always in danger of hurting the knee.

The slow running was easy on my knee, but hard on my self-
image. Trained on gut-tearing workouts with hard intervals and dry
heave recoveries, I didn't feel like a runner anymore. It took a few
months of ambling around the streets and parks of Berkeley before I
could hear, "Hey, you're breaking the speed limit!" or, "Mommy,
lookit the jogger!" without wincing.

And by the time I had developed "catcall calmness," I didn't
need it anymore. By that time, my endurance range had expanded
so much that I ran up into the hills and beyond, on untravelled roads
and trails, far from the jeers of slobs. Here I was alone, except for the
occasional runner in search of the same quiet solitude. Whenever I
came across someone going in my direction, we would while away
the miles in casual conversation. It was in one of these chance meet-
ings that I talked with my first real, live marathoner.

"You say you run marathons," I said. "What's it like? What
does it take to hold up over that distance? Twenty-six miles sounds
unreal to me, like a myth or a legend."

"Well," he said. "You say you run up to 15 miles on weekends.
That's not too hard on you, is it? You could run a marathon if you
wanted to. All you have to do is slow down and spread your energy
out over a longer distance and time. It's not an impossible feat, you
know."

"Are you serious?" I said. "Do you really think I could run one?"

He laughed. "Why not? I can tell you're in better shape than I am. If you're really interested, I've got a couple of entry blanks to the Golden Gate marathon. It's a beautiful course. I'm sure you'll enjoy yourself."

Two weeks later, I was caught up in the early morning excitement of my first road race. Runners were jogging around nervously, or taping their toes, or smearing vaseline over their feet. Everyone seemed to know everyone else, as if they belonged to a big happy family. My friend introduced me to Bob Deines, one of the runners described in the LSD book.

"Bob has been having problems ever since his last 50-miler. He's just going the first 10 miles as an easy workout. Why don't you run with him?"

"What pace are you planning, Bob?" I asked him.

"Slow training pace, somewhere between 7:30 and 8:00 per mile. If this is your first marathon, it might be a good idea to start with me."

Bob and I waited for the gun at the back of the pack. We let everyone get ahead, and loafed along at a conversational pace, paying more attention to a discussion of training methods than to the way the race was unfolding. At 10 miles, Bob dropped out. The time was 74 minutes (7:24 pace).

"I'm going to catch a ride to the 20-mile mark in Sausalito," he said. "Keep the pace down and you should be all right."

By now, I was beginning to think that I might manage the whole distance. The pace felt easy, and I was enjoying the role of "California distance runner." I was enormously proud of the number pinned on the front of my singlet. By the time I came into Sausalito, it was disintegrating with sweat and I had to stuff it into the waistband of my shorts. That made me feel like a seasoned veteran. The 20-mile point came shortly before the long climb up to the Golden Gate bridge. Bob Deines shouted out my time for me.

"You're right on pace, 2:30. Joe Henderson's about 200 yards ahead of you. See if you can catch him."

I felt really strong at that point. As I came up behind Joe, I wanted to thank him for the changes his book had made in my life, but he was talking to another runner. I didn't want to interrupt, so I kept going.

"Not even breathing hard," I said to myself. "He must be taking it easy."

I pushed hard up the hill and over the windy bridge. Coming
down the road to the Marina Greens was like flying, but when I hit
the flat section leading to the finish chute, it was all I could do to
keep my legs turning over.

I finished 71st, in 3:14:21. Drained of energy, I wandered
around in a happy daze. I was still in a daze as I watched the awards
ceremony. The winner was Rich Delgado, with a time of 2:31-some-
thing. As he carried away his trophy, I reflected that he had run
some 44 minutes faster than I had—almost two minutes per mile faster. It was staggering. I doubted my ability to run a single mile at his
pace, let alone 26 of them. But the comparison took nothing from
my personal victory. Finishing the distance was more than enough
for me.

I noticed with surprise that the old "not tough enough" feeling
was no longer there. I didn't know if it was the casual atmosphere of
that particular race, or the atmosphere of road running in general.
Somehow the rough and ready randomness of the roads gave me a
freedom that the clean precision of a 440 track denied me.

I rested for a few days after that race, and when I got out on
the roads and trails again, I started going longer than before. But the
pace remained slow and comfortable. I made sure I finished each run
with the feeling (often illusory I am sure) that I could repeat the distance without strain.

8 Two Racing Break Throughs

"On action alone by thy interest," said the Bhagavad Gita, "never on its fruits. Let not the fruits of action be thy motive." As I ran up into the Berkeley hills one morning, it occurred to me that my running was beginning to reflect those lines. In high school and college, my interest had been on the "fruits"—on good racing performance and the self-respect that they would have earned me. When I had been swimming, and even when I had started with slow running, my interest had still been on the "fruits" of activity, although now it was health rather than competition.

Watching my steamy breath, listening to the crunching of the frosty trail underfoot, feeling the warmth in my working muscles—that's where my interest was. I had no ambitions about racing, and I had long ago stopped worrying about maintaining health. What I was really interested in, what I really loved, was the running itself. Realizing that gave me a peaceful glow inside.

As I came off the last steep section and settled into the long winding flat section, I saw another runner ahead of me. He looked vaguely familiar, even at a distance from behind. His style was smooth and economical. His pace was a little slower than mine. He smiled a greeting as I came up alongside him.

"Do you mind if I run along with you for a while," I said.

"Not at all. I'd be glad for some company and conversation."

We ambled along easily. I sensed that he was holding enormous power in check.

"Is this your usual training pace?" I asked him.

"It has been for a few months. When I'm in shape I go faster, but right now I'm coming back from a bad case of mono I had last summer."

We ran comfortably to the end of the fire trail, where it joins the road.

"I usually turn around here," I said. "Thanks for the company, Maybe I'll see you again some time."

"I'll run back along the flat part of the trail," he said. "I want to get a few more miles in today. Do you mind if we pick it up a little?"

"Depends what you mean by a little," I said. "I'll try to stay with you. Don't let me hold you back."

His idea of a little was my idea of a lot. Within a half-mile, we were going so fast I had to bring my attention completely into the movement—the stride, the footfall, the arm swing, the breathing. There was such beautiful fluid power in his running that I got caught up in it, and swept along with it.

And he pushed the pace up, slowly and steadily. Every now and then I had a fleeting moment of panic. "I'm way out of my depth. Can I hold out to the next bend? Can I even hold out to that tree trunk?" But if I forgot my fears and let myself be carried along by the flow of his energy, suddenly it was easy and I was thinking, "Of course I can do it. All I have to do is let myself go."

That drive lasted for about two miles, the fastest two miles I had ever run in my life. When we slowed to a trickling jog just before the trail plunged down into Strawberry Canyon, I was astonished. I would never have believed myself capable of such sustained speed.

"That was an incredible run," I said when I had my breath back under control. "Thanks a lot for setting the pace."

"I should be thanking you," he answered. "I thought you were setting the pace. I haven't run that fast in a long time."

I knew he was just trying to make me feel good, but I wasn't going to turn down a compliment. Besides, I could read genuine gratitude in his eyes. Maybe I *had* helped him simply by hanging on.

"Do you want to run together next weekend?" he said. "We could meet at the bottom of the trail. I'm usually there at about eight o'clock."

"Sure," I said. "I'd love to. By the way, my name's Ian Jackson."

We shook hands as a mere formality. We had already met each other on that fast drive.

"I'm glad we ran into each other. My name's Rich Delgado."

First it was one day on the weekends, then both days, then early mornings during the week too. We got into the habit of daily runs together. Other runners joined us, some on weekends, some in the weekday mornings, some every day. But the core of the group was the relationship between Rich and I.

There was something about running with him that set me free from all my old performance hangups. For the most part, we ran pure LSD, but occasionally, when the mood was right, we got into long fast runs, playing with incredible speed.

I never knew how it happened. We would be easing along at 7:00 per mile and one of us (I never knew which one) would surge very slightly. Then we'd both be onto the pace of the surge. Later, there'd be another surge—just a little, almost unnoticeable increase in pace. But we kept pushing it up. Once we were moving, we didn't back off. Back and forth we'd play with the pace. He'd throw in a little more tempo. I'd match it and throw in a little of my own. Within a mile we'd go from 7:00 down to 6:30 pace. Two miles later, we'd be under 6:00. Another mile and we'd be down to about 5:30. It was so smooth you hardly knew it was happening. Finally, we'd be flying at 5:15 or 5:10, and the miles would reel by effortlessly.

There was something liberating in the knowledge that we could back off at any time. We weren't in pursuit of the leaders. We weren't in flight from the chasers. We were simply doing what felt good. Since I hadn't set the pace as a test of myself, there was nothing to prove, and, with nothing at stake, I could relax at speed.

I took this relaxed attitude with me into two breakthrough races—the Magnan cross-country run at Woodside (about 16 miles that year) and the West Valley marathon in Burlingame.

I started out very easily in the Magnan race. It took me about six miles to work my way up to Rich, running his first serious race since coming down with mono.

"How are you feeling?" I asked him.

"Worried about that hill," he said.

Following his eyes, I saw in the distance a broad cut up the side of a high ridge. It looked straight up and down. I widened my eyes in mock disbelief. He nodded with a grim smile.

By the time we had labored to the top of that muddy mountain, we were in third and fourth place. Coming out at the top, we passed Jose Cortez. The guides had not yet arrived at the ridge road, so he was feverishly making direction arrows out of branches.

We ran south on the ridge road and then turned down a trail that led back to Woodside. At the head of the trail, Rich was fighting a sideache. He told me to go ahead. "You might win this race," he said.

Ian Jackson at the finish of the 1972 West Valley Marathon. Time: 2:33:05. Joyful running. "I just took a back seat, concentrated on keeping the running body in precise trim, and let the energy express itself."

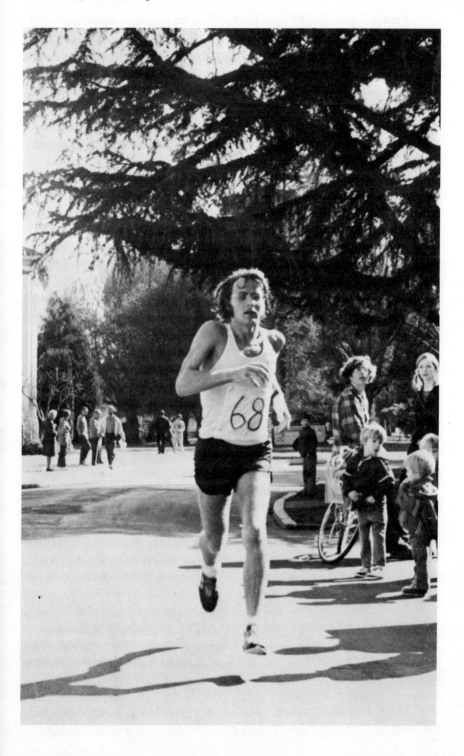

I surged and caught up with the leader, Duncan Macdonald. "We might be able to come in one-two-three for West Valley Track Club," I told him. "Rich is right behind us. If I can stay with you we've got it made."

"You stay with me?" he said. "I'll be lucky if I can stay with you."

That turned me on. Duncan Macdonald, a sub-four-minute miler, was worried about staying with me. I picked up the pace and he fell back. Now I was leading. I had all the energy in the world. All the runners behind me were pushing me along. The sensation of being out front was intoxicating.

Then Jose Cortez caught me. We exchanged grins as he went by. I felt warmth for him because of the personal style he had shown in stopping to mark the trail. He hadn't let the thrill of leading block his sense of responsibility to the other runners. I didn't think I could match his pace, so I let him go. I didn't want to get into the old pattern of "Why don't I have the guts to stay with him?" If I had tried to hang on, I might have surprised myself, but I was so enjoying the feel of my running body that I didn't want to risk spoiling it.

I finished second, pretty close behind Jose. The rest of the field was well behind us. That race was intensely exciting, and so was the West Valley marathon.

In the marathon, which was nine months after my initial 3:14 effort, I felt that same joy in running. Again, I started slowly, and took the first few miles to work myself into a state of passive attentiveness. I forgot about actively striving to compete with the other runners, and simply focussed on technical perfection—smooth stride, light foot placement, relaxed body carriage, balanced arm swing, rhythmic breathing, and other details.

I forgot about effort. I just took a back seat, concentrated on keeping the running body in precise trim, and let the energy express itself. My five-mile split was a personal record, as were the 10-, 15-, 20- and 25-mile splits. And yet I felt as if I was getting a free ride. The pace seemed an easy jog.

The first 12 finishers broke 2:30. I came in 13th at 2:33:05. Rich didn't run that race, but he was just as excited as I was about my time. "You're not far off the Olympic Trials qualifying time," he said. "I know you're capable of a sub-2:30. It's just a matter of time and training."

I was so amazed that a no-talent runner like me could race competently on primarily slow training that I began reading all I could find on the endurance method. The best source of information was the work of Dr. Ernst van Aaken, a German sports doctor who recommends plenty of aerobic endurance running, getting the body weight down and going on regular fasts to teach the body to live off its reserves.

I read about one of van Aaken's proteges, a top German marathoner by the name of Meinrad Nagele. At age 37, Meinrad was overweight and out of shape. At age 46, he ran a 2:29 marathon, finishing fourth in the World Veterans championship. After that race, he wrote, "The vast improvement I attribute to endurance training carried out consistently over a period of many years, together with a special diet (involving natural foods and fasting). This combination is the only method guaranteed to permit acquisition of the highest possible endurance potential."

I was immediately intrigued. What would happen if I combined Meinrad's "special diet" with the running I was already doing? Maybe I could become a really outstanding runner. After all the years of carrying the failure image, it was an exciting possibility.

9 Yes, I'm the Great Pretender

A special diet. Natural foods and fasting. I'd never heard much about either before, so I plunged enthusiastically into anything I could find on the subjects. And I started experimenting. Because it was unusual, I tried fasting first. For four consecutive weeks, I ate my last meal on Thursday night, fasted all day Friday, took my usual long run on Saturday morning and broke the fast after the run.

These first fasts were experimental. I felt generally comfortable throughout, aside from very brief periods of weakness and vague hints of headache. Running was easy, both on the regular Friday morning distance and the long Saturday morning explorations. I was so relaxed throughout the fasts that I decided to try an extra day.

On the fifth trial, I didn't break my fast after the long Saturday run. I took another long run on Sunday, and it was such a pleasant "floating" run that I decided to fast on Monday, too. In the early morning, as I started out on the usual "collection circuit" to pick up the others, I was moving at a shuffle. I almost gave up on the run so that I could go back for breakfast and some energy. But as the other runners joined me and warmed into the usual pace, I had no trouble staying with them. By the time we met Rich Delgado, who was at the end of the circuit, fatigue was the farthest thing from my mind. By then, I was totally turned on by the sheer pleasure of running.

That taught me how much of fatigue is mental. Morning after morning it was the same—a lethargic shuffle for the first couple of miles. Then, as other runners joined me and the pace slowly got faster, the energy came. I felt strong through the rest of the run, and through the rest of the day.

I kept on the fast for seven full days. On the last day, I had a peak experience. From the first steps, I was in a state of calm awareness. I was thinking about the "impossibility" of running almost 20 miles a day for seven days of fasting, but I was aware of the thought without being attached to it. I was also aware of the effortless glide—smooth, mellow and peaceful. I watched the pace creep up as, one after the other, we threw in subtle surges.

Cold air on the skin, fast footfalls, rhythmic breathing. We flew through drifting mist, in a forest of dark wet tree trunks and down-trailing branches. The gentle wind in the trees, the creaking of branches, the clear bird calls—all seemed to echo in the chambers of my heart. My very skin seemed to have opened up so that the energy of the universe could play within me, in the emptiness between the whirling atoms. Filled with elation and gratitude, I watched my body move on.

Even when we ran the long steep hills out of Tilden Park, I felt no effort. My body seemed somehow insubstantial, like some ethere-al vehicle of awareness. Running at speed was as easy as imagining it.

I wish I had continued with that fast. I broke it because the old conditionings about food were beginning to worry me: "You must have food, you know," "You'll starve within three or four days," etc. I have had other peak experiences during subsequent long fasts, but none has approached the intensity and peace of the first one.

As for natural foods, I read extensively in the field, most of it poorly written, sensational nonsense. The best sources were the hy-gienists—the European Are Waerland (Meinrad Nagele's mentor) and the American Herbert Shelton. Shelton was a rare find. If I had read him before learning how wrong established wisdom can be, I probably would have dismissed him as a faddist.

But I was more open to unconventional ideas now. Besides, reading Shelton was like being inside a strong mind as it analyzed and synthesized a complex problem. Although his beliefs were so startling as to sound dogmatic and uninformed, he introduced them by giving full attention to the relevant facts. I especially liked the way he quoted generously from sources that challenged his ideas. He would never say simply "This is wrong." He would instead explore the ob-jections with thoroughness so that you were with him when he said, "This doesn't account for these facts." Reading his books showed me the excitement of independent thinking. It prepared me to accept the attitude of the motto of his *Hygienic Review:* "Let us have truth, though the heavens fall." From a psychological point of view, his writing was a liberation.

And from a physical point of view, it was a source of unprece-dented vitality. On the hygienic diet—fresh fruits and vegetables, with nuts as the main source of protein—I felt my energy levels climb-ing steadily, just when I needed more energy to keep up with Rich.

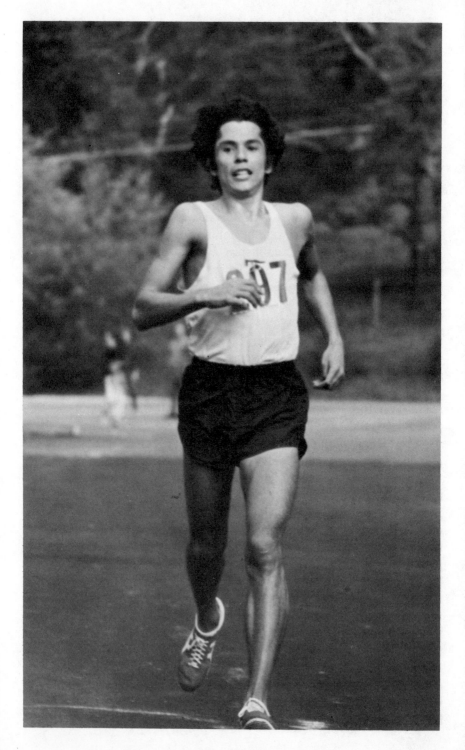

"Don't expect to stay with him when he gets back in shape," my
running friends had told me. "He had to lay off after coming down
with mono, but before that he had 12 years of pretty solid running.
You won't be able to train with him when he builds up his strength
again."

Not be able to train with him? No more running with Rich?
That meant I wouldn't be able to fly with him on those playful speed
runs. I'd have no one to help me train down to a sub-2:30. No more
witty miles of verbal fencing. I'd be falling behind again as I had in
school racing, falling behind and blaming myself for it. I couldn't
let that happen.

I convinced myself that a fast marathon time was the most important thing in the world. I pretended that I wanted to use myself as another Meinrad Nagele—to succeed in running with the help of natural
foods and fasting. It was only later, when yoga had put me in touch
with my feelings, that I was able to see into the heart of the matter.
Then I realized the depth of the emotional relationship developed over
those thousands of miles of running. Rich was moving away from me
in physical condition, and I wanted to stay with him not so much because it would improve my running as because it would keep me in emotional contact with him.

For a while, the extra vitality from the special diet was enough.
As Rich got stronger, and the runs increased in speed and distance, I
felt myself being carried along by an enormous wave of organic power.
For several months, I amazed myself day after day, matching him
stride for stride on runs far more demanding than any race. There
was so much at stake that I *had* to excel myself. But even the best of
diets cannot support continual overstress. Eventually, I began to
break down. In helpless misery, I felt myself slipping back. It was
all the more agonizing because I refused to face the truth.

Rich noticed my difficulties, and he was very considerate. When
I couldn't stay with him on the hills, he'd circle around at the top till
I joined him. When I couldn't keep up my end of the speed play on
the flat, he'd stop pushing the pace up, or even let it drift down a
little.

I just wasn't strong enough to stay with him, not tough enough.
I began to notice slight but persistent leg pains, mostly in the hamstrings. To ease off until the pains died down was unthinkable, because then I'd fall even further behind. So I kept running.

**Rich Delgado, Northern California Runner of the Year in 1970. "There
was such beautiful fluid power in his running that I got caught up in it,
and swept along by it." (John Marconi photo)**

I became a fine technician in what could be called stylistic bandaging. I learned to run delicately around the pain by playing with footfalls, knee lifts, back kicks, body carriage and other adjustments. Somehow, I was always able to find the right running motion to reduce the pain. I got pretty good at ignoring what I couldn't refine out.

Although my legs were always aching, although they kept me awake at night, I forced myself to keep running. And the pains got progressively worse. Finally, I had to start making excuses. I'd talk about having to study for language proficiency exams or for comprehensives. I'd say I had research work to do on a seminar paper. The real reason for skipping occasional runs, or for going slowly by myself, was rest and recuperation. Maybe I'd be able to run at Rich's level again if I could only get some time for recovery.

We went to races together, but I was no longer competitive. Runners who had never challenged me before were now beating me with ease. Then, two races in a row, I disgraced myself by dropping out. Even in the worst of my school races, I had never done that.

I still had enough common sense left to realize I was overstressed, but I didn't know enough about stress to make corrections. Remembering that Hans Selye's work had been cited in support of LSD training, I bought a copy of his brilliant book, *The Stress of Life*. In one sitting I read it from cover to cover, with the growing excitement of increasing clarity.

As I read Selye, I heard echoes of Shelton's ideas. Since I had been interested only in what Shelton had to say on natural foods and fasting, I had glossed over his repeated warnings against taking a part of the hygienic living instead of embracing it whole. Exercise is not enough, diet is not enough, fasting is not enough, fresh air and sunshine and pure water are not enough, nor are rest and sleep, nor is emotional poise. In order to live hygienically, that is, naturally, according to the laws of physiology, the whole lifestyle must be properly ordered. Shelton emphasized that unnatural living habits were a drain on the nervous system, and that impaired health was the inevitable consequence of insufficient nervous energy.

Selye focussed on the glandular system rather than the nervous system, but his insights were basically the same. He spoke of our inheritance of a certain amount of "adaptation energy," and the remarks about this energy were parallel to Shelton's remarks about vitality, or nervous energy.

Selye said that adaptation energy is like "a special kind of bank account which you can use up by withdrawals but cannot increase by deposits." He spoke of the two forms in which this energy is stored. There is "the superficial kind, which is ready to use; and the deeper kind, which acts as a kind of frozen reserve. When superficial adaptation energy is exhausted through exertion, it can slowly be restored from a deeper store during rest. This gives a certain plasticity to our resistance. It also protects us from wasting adaptation energy too lavishly in certain foolish moments, because acute fatigue automatically stops us."

"Experiments on animals have clearly shown that each exposure (to excess stress) leaves an indelible scar, in that it uses up reserves of adaptability which cannot be replaced. It is the restoration of superficial adaptation energy from the deep reserves that tricks us into believing that the loss has been made good. Actually, it has only been covered from reserves—and at the cost of depleting reserves. We might compare this feeling of having suffered no loss to the careless optimism of a spendthrift who keeps forgetting that whenever he restores the vanishing stocks of dollars in his wallet by withdrawing from the invisible stocks of his bank account, the loss has not really been made good. There was merely a transfer of money from a less accessible to a more accessible form."

The thought that I was squandering irreplaceable life energy through severe overstress was disturbing enough to make me reorder priorities. Selye's work made me see that I was dealing with ultimate questions about the value of life itself. He formulated the natural aim for man: it should be "to express himself fully, according to his own lights."

"The goal is certainly not to avoid stress," he said. "Stress is a part of life. It is a natural by-product of all our activities. There is no more justification for avoiding stress than for shunning cold, exercise, or love. But in order to express yourself fully, you must first find your ultimate stress level, and then use your adaptation energy at a rate and in a direction adjusted to the innate structure of your mind and body. It is not easy . . . It takes much practice and almost constant self-analysis."

That did it. I had been reluctant about missing runs and going slowly by myself. Now I took it easy with few qualms. Once you have seen clearly that overtraining is wasting your own life energy, moderation comes naturally.

10 The Laziness of Yoga

Just when I needed it, I read Joe Henderson's article, "The Runner's Final Stretch" in *Runner's World*. It explained why my legs hurt so much, and suggested how to ease the present pain and prevent future pain—by regular stretching.

For Joe, running was natural smooth movement. Exercise was "funny, phony, jerky little dances inflicted as punishment by army drill sergeants and done in desperation by overweight housewives."

But running had become increasingly difficult for him. "Right now, my left heel hurts like hell. It has been hurting like that for the last seven or eight months. For several months before that, my right achilles tendon was messed up. Before that, my right calf muscle was pulled. There have been other things."

He had decided to look for medical help. The podiatrist quickly found out what was wrong.

"Your calves are unusually strong and tight, even for a runner," he said. "You're overdeveloped there from your years of running. Your achilles tendon is like a rubber band that is always stretched to the point of breaking. When you put the slightest extra pull on it, something gives. Sometimes it's the achilles itself, sometimes the calf muscle. In this case, it's the area where the tendon attaches to the heel. Unless you do something about those tight calves, you'll keep having trouble."

Once he knew the problem, the solution fell into place.

Joe told his office mate, George Beinhorn, about the tightness. "The only thing the guy didn't tell me was what to do about it." George didn't tell him either. He showed him. He got out of his chair and slapped his palms flat on the floor, stiff-kneed and without a warmup.

"We're running about the same mileage," George said. "But I do yoga, too. I don't get any injuries."

George Sheehan, medical editor of *Runner's World*, shared Joe's problems. "I think LSD, with its tight economical little stride, promotes tight hamstrings, calves and achilles. I started some yoga and flexibility exercises, and I thought it would tear my muscles apart. I'm too impatient to keep at it, but in your case it must be done."

Finally, Joe came across an article in *Fitness for Living* magazine— "Stretch those Muscles!" According to the author, Robert Bahr, most active people ignore the need for flexibility. "Strengthening and endurance exercise, while essential to total fitness, nonetheless acts to shorten muscles and reduce flexibility . . . Most cases of muscle tears and pulls and strains occur because of lack of flexibility."

Bahr quoted Dr. Herbert H. de Vries to support his position: "Stretching by jerking, bobbing or bouncing methods (as in calisthenics) invokes the stretch reflexes, which actually oppose the desired stretching." And he gave his layman's interpretation: ". . . when a muscle is jerked into extension, the natural reaction is for the muscle to jerk back, thus shortening itself again. But when the stretch is achieved slowly and held for a period of time, another reaction takes place . . . which helps relax the muscle being stretched."

Joe's article was illustrated with photos of Robert Bahr doing some simple stretching exercises. They looked easy, but when I tried them I thought, like George Sheehan, that they "would tear my muscles apart."

I was so tight that when I tried to touch my toes, I could barely reach midway between my knees and the floor. Bahr's exercises did not appeal to me, so I went out and bought a few yoga books to learn from.

I started with Richard Hittleman's *Be Young With Yoga.* I liked Hittleman's book because the yoga poses (asanas) were demonstrated by Hittleman's students—housewives, school teachers and businessmen. If they could do it, so could I. Besides, the book presented a manageable seven-week course. I assumed I would be loose and flexible as soon as I had paid my seven weeks' dues. It was an attractive goal to look forward to.

But I soon found that the yoga poses were not very different from Bahr's exercises. When I tried to do them, I still felt as if I was tearing my muscles apart. But I wanted badly to get back into running, so I forced myself hard. I hoped that my muscle tightness would be as easy to work out as it is to break up encrusted mud on a running shoe. Surely a few of the right twists and flexes would get things loosened up, I thought.

After a week of excruciating self-torture, my leg pains were worse than before. I decided that this yoga stuff was not what it was made out to be. Hittleman claimed that once you've learned how to do hatha yoga, "you will find that you will never want to give it up."

Not only did I *want* to give it up, I was suffering so much that I *had* to give it up.

I took a week's rest to recuperate, reread the instructions more attentively and then started in again, much more gently and carefully this time. The relaxed approach made all the difference: I began to understand Hittleman's claim.

Within five months, I was reasonably adept with the asanas in his seven-week course, and I started to look for something more challenging. Searching in the local bookstores, I found a silver-covered paperback called *Light on Yoga,* by B.K.S. Iyengar. As I looked through the hundreds of photographs, I was awestruck. Iyengar's asanas had a poignant, unearthly beauty in them. They made my heart swell with the sweet ache of loneliness. I didn't realize it at the time, but I had discovered the modern classic of hatha yoga.

I forgot Hittleman and plunged right into the 300-week course outlined in Iyengar's book. It was like jumping from the jogging program at the local YMCA straight into an Olympic training camp with Lydiard, Bowerman or van Aaken. Working without a teacher was difficult. Had I not had those five months of easy introduction, I would have given up.

After a few weeks, I dropped all pretenses of running. Iyengar-style yoga was totally engrossing. I didn't need anything else. I might easily have become another stale running dropout.

But yoga kept pushing me back. As I became loose and flexible, my body began to feel "weightless." Movement became a sensual pleasure. I started running again because it excited me again. The sensation of light-footedness or "light-bodiedness" was delightful.

When I had been working with Iyengar's book for about a month, I got a call from Bob Anderson at World Publications. For well over a year, ever since finding out about *Runner's World,* I had been asking him about a job whenever I was down by the office.

"We've got an opening in layout," Bob said. "I know that's not your bag, but if you're really interested, the job could be a foot in the door for you."

Persistence had paid off. "When do I start?" I asked.

Since Mountain View was too far away for commuting, I would have to move down there, away from my wife. That might have stood in the way, but we had been talking about separation anyway, and the job gave us an excuse to live apart without as much personal sting as there would have been without it.

As Bob had said, layout was not my bag, but it did open up many opportunities for writing. When he was working on the *Exercises for Runners* booklet, Joe Henderson asked me if I'd like to do the yoga section.

"I don't know of any runners who are more into yoga than you are," he said. "I think our readers would find your experiences interesting."

So I wrote an enthusiastic article about my pathway to Iyengar's book, and I added a section of photos describing the asanas I was working on. By this time, I was even more excited about the Iyengar method. I tried hard to get in touch with him, with no success. The publishers of *Light on Yoga* ignored my letters, and the yoga teachers I asked all knew about him, but not his whereabouts.

"Iyengar is an absolute terror," one teacher told me. "He's also an absolute genius. There's no one I'd rather study under. Someone told me he has an institute in London. If I had the money, I'd be in England with him right now."

No one could give me any better information. I had almost given up hope when I heard of a South African couple living in nearby Palo Alto—Felicity and David Hall. I was told that David was a research engineer in computer science at the Stanford Research Institute. He had delivered a paper on yoga and computer science at a yoga conference in India. Felicity had been a yoga teacher for five years, and was one of the few teachers in the country working with Iyengar's methods. She went to France each year to study with J.B. Rishi, one of Iyengar's longtime students. But I didn't have to go to England or France or India; contacting her was as easy as consulting the phone book. Her accent told me I had the right number.

I told her about my yoga background, and about my article on Iyengar.

"I'm on the 30th week of his course right now," I said.

"If you're that advanced, I don't think I can teach you anything," she said. "If you're interested, though, you're welcome to the class. We meet at seven tonight."

Hungry for approval, I took the exercise booklet along with me. She seemed very pleased to see it, but she scrutinized the photos for an uncomfortably long time. The verdict hung in suspense.

"These are not too bad," she said. "The mistakes are not likely to mislead your readers. Iyengar himself will be interested in this. He's going to be in the San Francisco area in about a month for a teacher training seminar."

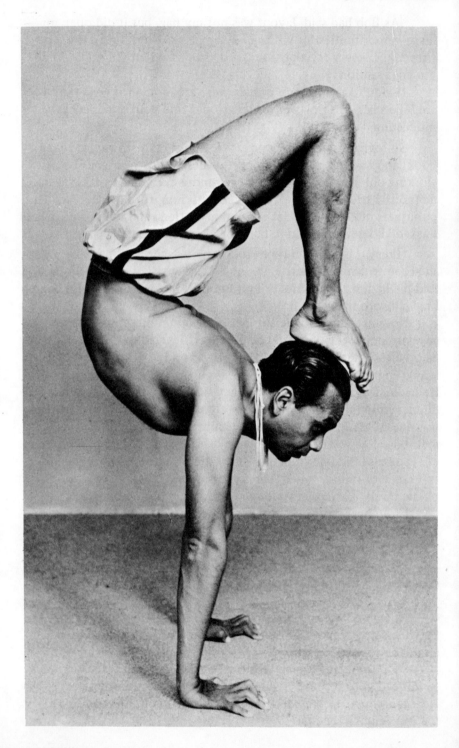

"Iyengar's coming here? In person?" I couldn't believe my
ears. "I've just got to attend that seminar. Is it too late to get in?"
"The class was overfull long ago," she said. "And there's already
a waiting list. I'll see if I can help you out."
She did manage to secure me a place in the seminar, and in the
weeks leading up to it, she helped me refine the poses I had demonstrated so clumsily in the yoga booklet.

The tension was stifling. There was no escape now. Iyengar
glided into the hall like a stalking panther. Fierce eyes, silver hair,
flowing white robe on dark skin. In aching silence, with breathtaking
grace, he unbuttoned. He was wearing a pair of trunks and a singlet.
As he walked to the stage, his bare feet rang authority on the hardwood floor. His predatory eyes surveyed us. Three rows of cross-
legged anticipation.
"I can see by the way you're sitting that none of you know
what yoga is," he said. "Yoga is one, but your postures tell me that
you believe in different yogas—bakti yoga, jnana yoga, karma yoga,
and the yoga you hope to learn from me: hatha."
"Teachers get drunk with ego," he continued. "In the next
three days, you will taste the water of humility again. Now you will
learn how to stand. Get up. Kick your mats against the wall."
He demanded unwavering attention. Lapses were punished by
resounding cuffs and slaps. I got more than my fair share. My neck
and shoulders were tight and I couldn't release them.
"Relax your brain!" he shouted at me. "Relax your neck, relax
your throat, relax your tongue. Stiff neck, sore brain. You cannot
think with a stiff neck. You cannot run."
When he was satisfied, he jumped up on the stage and surveyed
us intently. I felt strange—detached and involved at the same time.
"The books all say that bakti yoga is pure devotion and hatha is
pure body. But are you not showing pure devotion right now in the
way your feet kiss the ground?"
His question shocked me. At that very moment I was feeling
solidly balanced, totally relaxed, and marvelously alert. The very
cells of my body seemed aware. My fear of Iyengar was nothing com-
pared to the joy that buoyed me.

**B. K. S. Iyengar, master teacher and author of Light on Yoga. "The
way I am teaching, you become the full moon, ever bright, ever active,
ever throwing light and joy to the world." (photo courtesy of B. K. S.
Iyengar)**

"Put the brain in the body," he said. "Do not try to do the poses with the brain in the head. The muscles have their own intelligence."

He called us up to the stage to show us what he meant. For the sake of demonstration, he used the pose on page 66 (Uttitha Parshvakonasana).

"The forward leg must be at a right angle," he said. "The weight must go through the center of the shin bone. The slightest deviation forces the muscles to make compensations and counter-compensations. Watch the mistakes."

He smoothed the hair on the thigh of the forward leg, and went down into the pose with too much knee bend. The hairs stood on end. He smoothed them again and went into the pose with too little knee bend. Again they stood on end. Finally, he smoothed the hair and executed the pose correctly. This time the hairs remained smooth.

"All the books say that yoga is gentle and easy," he said. "They do not know. This is a strenuous pose, is it not? Yet my muscles are at ease. This is the art of true laziness in yoga."

I immediately remembered an account of a similar kind of laziness. In *Hara: The Vital Center in Man,* Karlfried Durckheim gives this example:

"Kenran Uneji, the archery master, bade his pupils test his arm muscles at the moment when his bow was drawn to its fullest extent— a bow which nobody but himself was able to draw. His muscles were completely relaxed. He laughed and said, 'Only beginners use muscle power—I draw simply with the spirit.'"

Iyengar demanded our complete attention, but he gave us far more than we could give him. In those three days, he worked tirelessly with us. His vitality was incredible. At age 56, he makes our strongest senior marathoners seem pallid in comparison. Rama Jyoti Vernon, the inspiration behind the California Yoga Teachers' Association, which sponsored Iyengar's visit, reported that he slept only four hours a night. "And yet he still runs us to a frazzle."

As he worked us in the poses, he dropped comments that helped my understanding of his approach. They were part of an ongoing flow of instruction, but they stood out for me.

"In practicing yoga," he said, "you learn to make friends with your body by exploring with clarity and courage... The moment you

believe you have perfected a pose, it becomes dead. Always work for
finer adjustments, always let the body continue to explore... You
have to be innocent to do yoga, you must be open to every experience
as it comes moment to moment. Without innocence you cannot feel
the fragrance of your action... You ask about sitting meditation? In
my opinion it is not necessary. Sitting meditation is like a sliver of the
moon. The way I am teaching, you become the full moon, ever bright,
ever active, ever throwing light and joy to the world. Sitting meditation quiets the mind. Yoga brings life to every cell in the body and
mind. It awakens you, it does not put you to sleep... The mind is a
dictator. Beginners in yoga always let the mind dictate to them. We
have to come to the point where the body says, 'You have dictated
for so long, now *I* am going to dictate. Can you obey me?' Watch for
that communication within yourself, then you have dialogue between
the body and the mind. It's like a change of government, a revolution."

I could only vaguely imagine what he was saying. At the time I
thought it was related in some way to listening to the body rather than
ignoring it as I had during my long bout of overtraining. It was about
six months later when I first began to feel the muscles "talking" to me,
and it was over a year before the body started dictating to the mind.
The catalyst for the final breakthrough was an outstanding teacher by
the name of Joel Kramer. But more of that in the last chapter.

11 Testing the Muscular Trap

I made rapid progress. Flexibility seemed to come easily. I noticed improvements even on a week-to-week basis. Then I started getting greedy. One day, when I was right on the edge of completing a twist pose, I strained to get all the way into it. Something snapped. A pulled back muscle.

I had been going to Felicity Hall's yoga class once a week. She sharpened my precision in the poses, and I worked on assimilating her instructions in my individual practice. The next night, my back was so painful I could barely draw a breath. I thought I might still be able to work on some standing poses, so I went to class in spite of the pain.

"What have you done to yourself?" asked Felicity as I walked into the room grimacing.

"Pulled a back muscle," I said. "At least I hope that's all I did."

"I worry about the way you push yourself. We all have a tendency to do it, but you more than others. Let's see if we can help relax the muscle with some very easy stretches."

"Would you like to try some Rolfing?" said David.

"Try what?"

"Rolfing. The technical name is structural integration. It's a form of deep massage developed by Ida Rolf. By direct work on the connective tissues, it aims to correct structural imbalance in the body. I can work on your back right now to see if we can straighten things out."

"Why not?" I said. "I'll try anything."

When David started working, I wished I'd kept my mouth shut. Using fingers and knuckles, he went deep and hard into the flesh. It hurt like hell.

"Don't hold your breath," he said. "Breathe into the pain as you would breathe into a yoga stretch."

That helped, but not much. I was thankful for the release from pain when he finished. I had forgotten all about the pulled muscle by then. The agony had completely masked it.

"Why don't you test it now," said David. "Try a gentle forward bend."

I eased gingerly into Paschimottanasana. There was no longer any pain. "I don't believe this," I said. "What did you do to me?" I could breathe deeply, I could twist, I could bend. "Whatever you did, thanks a lot."

By the time the class was over, I was aware of the muscle again, but only barely. I followed David and Felicity to their car, asking questions.

"I've got some literature in the glove compartment," David said. "If it interests you, you might also like the writings of Wilhelm Reich."

Most of the Rolf literature agreed with what I had read about the importance of good postural alignment for economical running:

"Because heads, shoulders, arms, etc., all have weight, a person standing must somehow support quite a load. He can do it basically in two ways. If the large bones in his body (tibia, femur, large lumbar vertebrae, etc.) are arranged with their centers of gravity one above the other (a plumbline dropped from the ear would pass through the shoulder, hip joint, knee, anklebone), those bones will serve as columns which will support the weight themselves. Very little muscular effort will be needed to keep the bones balanced that way, and all will be lovely. (Dr. Rolf likens this desirable situation to a set of children's blocks piled in the most stable way, with the center of gravity of each block directly over that of the one below.)

"On the other hand, the body's large bones may not normally be aligned in this stable way. The head may be thrust forward, for example, with the shoulders leaning back to compensate for it. The abdomen (and hence the lower spine) may be forward. (This is very common—take a close look at the next person you see standing in profile.) In that case enormous muscular effort must be expended just to prevent the whole wobbly tower from collapsing: the neck and upper back muscles must tighten to keep the head from falling to the chest, and so on down the body."

The body masses are rarely aligned well, because most of us have suffered various physical and psychological assaults which have molded our postures away from the ideal. The Rolfers have found that the release of the body masses from structural deformation "permits the emergence of a more sensitive being."

"Ancient mystery schools apparently understood this relation. There seems to be evidence that among their teachers were men expert in refining the body for the express purpose of furthering individual psychic progression. In some areas, remnants of this still survive. Witness the branch of yoga sometimes misnamed hatha.

"If done properly, most of these (hatha yoga) asanas seem to be powerful tools for moving the body toward the kind of balanced alignment Rolfers seek."

The first thing I read about Wilhelm Reich's work was *Me and the Orgone*, by TV personality Orson Bean. I enjoyed Bean's lively account of his first session of Reichian therapy.

His doctor was Ellsworth Baker (whose *Man in the Trap* was my next book). He explained to Dr. Baker that his life was not difficult in any way, but that "I would never be satisfied until I felt fulfilled and, dare I say it, really happy..."

Dr. Baker asked him to undress. "My eyes went glassy as I stood up..." He followed instructions dutifully "hoping to get a gold star." He felt strained and uptight. "What if I get an erection, or shit on his bed, or vomit?"

Baker began pressing and probing the tight muscles around Bean's neck and jaw. "Did that hurt?" he asked, and then, "Why didn't you cry?" Bean replied, "I'm a grown-up." Baker didn't let up, but continued to prod and probe. Bean began to let his feelings out a little. "I managed to let out a few pitiful cries which I hoped would break Baker's heart."

The pain was so intense that he "no longer worried about getting an erection, possibly ever, but the possibility of shitting on his bed loomed even larger."

After working on the front of his body, Baker had Bean turn over so that he could work on his back. Then he asked him to breathe and roll his eyes around without moving his head. Bean followed instructions, "feeling rather foolish but grateful that he was no longer tormenting my body... I began to feel a strange pleasurable feeling in my eyes..." Baker then had him raise his legs and do a bicycle kick. "On and on I went until my legs were ready to drop off. Then, gradually, it didn't hurt any more and that same sweet fuzzy sensation of pleasure began to spread through my whole body, only stronger."

"I was breathing more deeply than I ever had before and I felt the sensation of each breath all the way down past my lungs and into my pelvis... Finally, I knew it was time to stop. I lay there for how many minutes I don't know, and I heard his voice say, 'How do you feel?' "

"Wonderful," I said. "Is this always what happens?"

Reichian therapy is based on the theory that our character traits are reflected in areas of muscular rigidity and tightness in the body. Characteristics of timidity, for instance, might be reflected in chronically tight neck and shoulder muscles. A timid person holds himself all day as if expecting a blow. Fear of sexuality might be reflected by a withdrawn pelvis, which moves the sexual organs back, producing outthrust buttocks and an exaggerated curve in the lower back.

Rather than wasting time trying to unearth the causes of the timidity or sexual fear, the Reichian therapist goes directly to the tight muscles in which the traits are bound up. When the muscular tightness is released, the traits they reflect are dissolved. Once the neck muscles are relaxed, the timidity is replaced by self-confidence. Once the pelvic tightness is relaxed, sexual fears evaporate.

Orson Bean's feelings of pleasure were produced by muscular relaxation and the corresponding release of character blocks. The next day, he was still feeling good. "My body felt light and little ripples of pleasure rolled up and down my arms, legs and torso... I felt vaguely horny in a tender way." But towards the end of the day he fell into a state of panic.. "It was a different kind of dread... I felt like I...was starting to come apart. The anxiety was terrific and I was aware that I was involuntarily tightening up on my muscles, to hold myself together." The old tightness in the muscular tissues was beginning to reassert itself, and with it, the "uptight" character traits.

I talked to David Hall again at Felicity's next class.

"This stuff is really exciting," I said. "It seems to me that I've been doing the same in yoga by myself. Do you think it's possible to release muscular tension and achieve structural integration through yoga alone?"

"If you have an excellent teacher, it may be possible. But my limited experience suggests to me that there are some "knots" in the tissues that can be easily dissolved in Rolfing, although they have persisted through years of yoga stretching. Good yoga is a great help to structural integration, but there is a limit to what you can do by yourself."

"This reminds me of distance training," I said. "Distance runners traditionally take one very long run per week, usually at least twice their daily average. The long runs bring big gains in endurance, and the shorter runs consolidate the gains. Would you say that yoga is like the regular daily runs and Rolfing like the long runs that produce big gains?"

"I think that's an interesting comparison," David said, "There's a big difference between the extra long runs and the Rolfing, though. The large gains in Rolfing come from a series of very brief crises rather than a gentle, long lasting stress."

For quite some time, I had been feeling more at ease with myself, more spontaneous and honest in expressing my feelings, and generally confident and high-spirited. Now that I knew about the ideas of Rolf and Reich, I began to make connections between my yoga practice and my increasing feelings of openness.

One day in Felicity's class, I told David that I was getting more and more interested in Rolfing for myself.

"Are you sure you want to do it?" he said. "I don't think it's a decision to be taken lightly."

"Yes, I'm sure," I said. "I think I can attain the same results through yoga, but I'd like to accelerate the process."

"Tell you what," he said. "You've already reserved a space in the J. B. Rishi yoga seminar next month. Think about it till then, and if you still want to do it, we'll have the first session just before the seminar."

"I don't think I'm going to change my mind," I said. "I'm sure I'm still going to want to do it."

And I still did. Three weeks later, I met David in his office. I undressed, and lay on the massage table. I felt tense and worried. I was trying to decide how I should be acting.

"Don't let goal striving get in your way," said David. "If you're searching for something, you'll get trapped in the idea of searching. Just be aware. Don't be rigid in your expectations. Simply be here now."

The probing got painful, very painful. I couldn't stop myself wincing and flinching. I tried to relax, but my muscles had a will of their own, and they tightened against the pressure. I didn't notice any emotional release during the session, but something must have been going on, because I felt a rapid change within myself during the five days of the J.B. Rishi seminar.

12 Balancing and Blossoming

J. B. Rishi had been giving workshops and seminars ever since arriving from Paris several weeks before. Nevertheless, he had the same boundless energy that had impressed me in Iyengar. He was slightly built, about my own height, with a grizzly beard and an infectious smile. When Felicity Hall introduced us, she mentioned that he had been a runner in his school days.

In my bastard French and his bastard English, we immediately began to talk about running, sports and yoga. I told him about my marathoning ambitions and how they had led to breakdown.

"I understand," he said, "I think this is very common with athletes. I too have gone through it. Competition was for me too much a matter of ego, of winning honors, of conquering. I could not see it at the time, but it stunted my personality, and impoverished my spirit."

"How did yoga change things?" I asked.

"It happened without my expecting it. When I had been practicing for some time, the competitive desire simply gave way to the desire to use my body to maintain a certain beauty within.

"I trained and raced so hard that I drained my energy reserves. Like you, I broke down, physically and mentally. Competition made a tyrant out of an aspect of my personality. Yoga was like a midwife helping the birth of my inner being."

I liked the way he put it. "How would you describe the essence of yoga?" I said.

"I think it is the quality of attention," he said. "Sport based on the competitive drive is pure destruction. Competitive drives are like blinders that narrow the field of attention. But sport based on the criteria of beauty, balance and unfolding of the inner being is pure creation. This kind of sport is a form of yoga. There is something in it that is comparable to art."

"There are many similarities between running and yoga. For instance, rhythm is important in both. Once you have perfected the asanas, you can practice them in a certain combination and with a rhythm that prevents the development of fatigue. Even in a long and intense session there is no exhaustion.

"Avoiding over- and underextension is also important. If you underextend, you do not stretch the muscles. If you overextend, you damage them. In running, if you do too little, you do not improve. If you do too much, you damage the heart, the tissues, and the muscles.

"If you practice sport as yoga, as a way of becoming aware of the body, you can develop the kind of sensitivity a skilled surgeon has. Yoga also brings deep relaxation. It can be used to stabilize your energy before competition and after."

"Have you found yoga to be a help for any of your students who were athletes?" I said.

"Definitely," he said. "When undertaken in the spirit of yoga, training is the art of living. It elevates the quality of your life. The danger is that this kind of training inevitably produces success in competition, and then you can get lost in your ego. It can become powerful and dominant. When success comes, you must let it go. You must hold fast to the inner being and not get lost in the personality."

The inner being is one thing and the personality is another? Before getting into yoga, this distinction had always seemed blurred, perhaps nothing more than the wishful thinking of restless people who wanted life to be richer than they found it. But now things were clearing up. The inner being could be found in pure feelings, feelings coming from the muscles and joints, from the internal organs, and from interpersonal relationships. The personality could be found in any and all ways in which our upbringing diluted and distorted those pure feelings.

In a race, the inner being was in the sensations of the running body, the personality was in the "shoulds" that put us out of contact with those sensations—"I should be tough," "I should master this pain," and all the other orders we give our bodies when they are crying for relief from our effort. This really came clear when I had a few more Rolfing sessions, which dramatized for me what was already happening through my yoga practice.

The session David had given me before the Rishi seminar had dealt with many parts of the body. It was a kind of groundwork for the subsequent sessions.

The second session was mainly from the knees down. For the first few minutes, the work was so excruciating that I almost called a halt to the proceedings. David was watching my breathing and my grimacing.

"Are you a masochist?" he asked.

"Perhaps," I answered. "Why do you ask?"

"You are going through intense pain. That could mean that you want to feel pain, because you want to be punished for something. The next question is obvious. Why do you want punishment? What are you guilty about?"

The more I brought out into the open, the more the body sensations changed. What had been ragged agony became pure, smooth sensation. By the end of the session the feelings were actually becoming pleasurable.

The work in the third session was mainly in the sides. The most sensitive parts were the hips. I felt very squeamish about being touched near the genitals, but by the end of the session I really felt alive. Warm streaming sensations coursed through my body and centered in the pelvic region.

Next morning, however, I was depressed and anxious. Like Orson Bean after Baker's Reichian therapy, I found my body clamping down again. I began to spend more time with yoga, to help keep the muscles loose, and to encourage the free flow of feelings.

The fourth session was the first of three that focus on the pelvis. It was this session that got me solidly back into running. The work was on the insides of the legs and around the pelvic rim. The feelings were intensely sexual. I was worried that I would get an erection and I felt acutely uncomfortable about getting turned on by another man. I reassured myself that it was the Rolfing, not the man, that was turning me on, but the reassurance was hollow.

"This is interesting," said David. "The muscles behind your thigh should be free and separate parts of a cluster that works as a unit. But yours are all clumped together by adhesions, in both legs."

After breaking the clumps up, David had me try a bicycling motion with the legs. I could feel life within the inner spaces as never before. Suddenly I had an overwhelming desire to run.

"Now slowly get off the table and stand in front of the mirror," David said. "Let the muscles remain as relaxed as they are now."

I got off the table carefully as I could, but I couldn't stop the leg muscles from tensing as I took my weight on my feet.

"All that work down the drain," said David. "I spend more than an hour relaxing your legs and now you tighten them again."

"But how can I be any more relaxed than I am now? I've got to use the muscles to balance on my feet!"

"That's right," David said. "But you can use them without tensing them."

"You mean like Iyengar demonstrated at the seminar?" I said.

"Exactly," he said. "We'll have to work on it. You should be able to stand with no effort at all if your large bones are properly aligned. Your leg muscles should be soft, not hard like they are now."

He had me sit down on a stool. Then he held my head and began moving it in small circles. "Just imagine that your body is hanging down from your head. Let the spine follow the head without interfering."

I got into touch with the sensations.

"This is fantastic!" I said. "It's like my whole spine is a tube of living light, like a luminous snake living inside me. I have an internal vision of it as a cobra swaying in front of a snake charmer."

"Good," said David. "Now sway on your own. Get in touch with the way gravity pulls on your body masses. Get rid of the notion that you have to make an effort to sit up straight. The muscles will make all the adjustments necessary without your help. You don't have to throw in your two bits worth. Don't give yourself unnecessary work."

"That could be good advice for running a race," I commented.

"Now close your eyes and be aware of the feeling as I adjust your posture."

He moved me around gently, balancing me on my sitting bones. I let myself relax under his hands.

"How does that feel?" he said.

"It feels like I'm slumping, slouching. The image in my mind is a hunch-backed Bowery bum sitting like human wreckage on a curb."

"Open your eyes and look at yourself in the mirror."

I stared at myself in disbelief. My posture was perfect.

"How can this be? I feel that I could easily go to sleep in this position. I feel like I'm floating in gravity instead of having to fight it. I feel like a lazy good-for-nothing."

"You see how our society conditions us to make effort?" David said. "Unless we're uptight and striving, we feel that we're sinning in some way. We actually feel guilt at pleasure and ease. It sounds ridiculous, and it is. But it's true."

"You know something," I said. "I think I'm beginning to understand what the true laziness of yoga is all about."

When we got to the fifth session, which was the abdominal muscles, the sexual feelings were on my mind. Never before had I been able to admit such feelings, let alone discuss them openly.

"I think I was getting sexually turned on last time," I told him.

David appeared neither shocked nor disconcertingly interested. With either reaction, I would have regretted speaking out. He simply acknowledged the revelation without comment. He continued working in the comfortable silence. I started chuckling to myself.

"You know," I said. "Suddenly I feel enormously relieved. I just had a flash of memory from my childhood. I think I was about 15 at the time, and my brother was 12. Anyway, I remember putting my arm around his shoulder one day, and feeling fear and confusion when he wrenched himself violently away. 'What are you? Some kind of queer or something?' he said. My own kid brother! I had loved him and hated him, shared with him and competed with him. Suddenly, for no reason, my feelings for him were sordid and perverted. That was a major turning point. Since then, I've blocked my feelings toward men, and in doing that, I've crippled my ability to respond to women, too. I've been trapped in the notion that feelings are bad, and have to be kept under control."

"It's good you're getting free of that," said David.

He was working on the rectus abdominis muscle. I felt free enough to tell him that his touch sent light electric shocks down to my genitals.

"There's a great deal of tension here," he said. "There's a real psychological knot living in these muscles."

I continued discussing the genital flashes when I felt them. Somehow, open discussion took the charge of guilt away. Suddenly I noticed that the flashes were gone. I felt as if I had shrugged off a heavy suit of armor.

"Good," said David. "Your abdominals are relaxed now."

"It's the first time in my memory," I said. "They've always tightened up when anyone touched me in that area, male or female. I guess it was a defense against sexual feelings. It's funny how these things work. I'm only just beginning to see how far out of touch with feelings of all kinds my defenses have made me. And it's only now that I can see how needless the defenses are. I'm beginning really to lose my fear of feeling."

13 Maps for Exploration

When you try these asanas, you'll probably discover that you're
tighter than you thought. Don't despair. The tightness gives you a fas-
cinating terrain for exploration.

Stretch as far as you can, but don't strain beyond the stretch into pain. Yoga is not self torture. It is not a play in pain, but rather a
play in awareness. Take Paschimottanasana, for instance (page 77).
This pose is excellent for exploring stretch because you can adjust your
reach very finely when doing a sitting forward bend.

You might be able to reach down to your toes, or you might find
yourself with your hands on your knees. If you're as tight as I was
when I started two years ago, you'll probably be at the edge of your
stretch when your hands are midway between your knees and your toes.
But wherever you find the edge of your stretch, stay there. Don't try
to push past it in the mistaken belief that the closer you come to the
completed position, the closer you are to "real yoga."

The real yoga is in the awareness with which you play the edges
of your stretch. If you force yourself into pain, you might *look* more
adept, but adeptness in yoga has little to do with how the pose looks
from the outside. Rather, it is a matter of how awarely you feel it from
the *inside*, how finely you tune into the edges of your stretch. So in
Paschimottanasana, don't worry about how far the edges of your stretch
will let you reach, just go as far as you can as awarely as you can. Approach all the asanas with this attitude. When you learn to do this,
you'll find that the edges of your stretch move further out. Simple
awareness brings change.

Breathe through the nose at all times, and try to make a low hiss-
ing sound in the back of your throat as the air moves in and out. This
is the same sound deep sleepers make. I think it helps relaxation in
the poses because it is associated in the brain and nervous system with
the relaxation of deep sleep.

You can use the breath to help you play the edges of your stretch.
Hold your position on the inbreath and then test the edges on the outbreath. Or hold on the outbreath and test the edges on the inbreath,
whichever feels more natural.

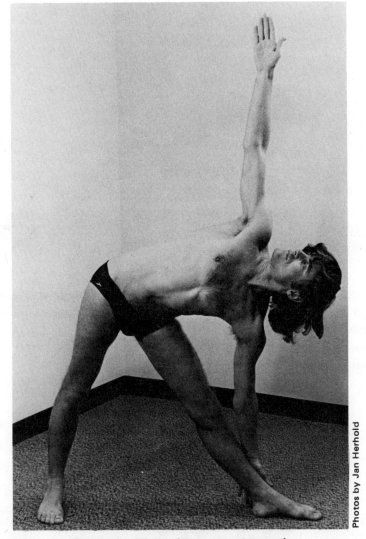

Photos by Jan Herhold

TRIKONASANA (The triangle pose)

You don't have to get your lower hand down to the floor. Staying within the limits of your stretch, bend to the side and rest your hand on your leg. Keep the kneecaps pulled up. Twist the body so that the lower ribcage comes forward and the upper ribcage moves back. Stretch the arms fully. Breath deeply and evenly. Hold the pose for one or two breaths at first. Slowly extend your endurance to half a minute to a minute.

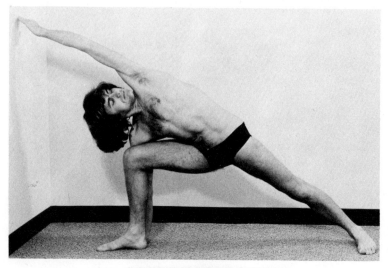

PARSHVAKONASANA

Feet are wider apart than in Trikonasana. The leg of the turned out foot is at a right angle. Although it is not necessary, I
have found it helpful to position myself so that I can stretch
for the wall with my upper arm as shown. I am a little too
close here; the wall should be about an inch out of reach.

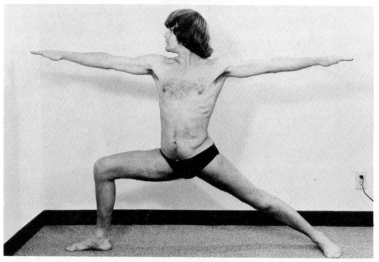

VIRABHADRASANA 1

Stretch out with the arms and up with the spine. I have found
it helpful to do this pose close up to a wall so that the backs
of my outstretched arms lie against the wall. I try to press
both buttocks *and* the outside of the bent knee to the wall.

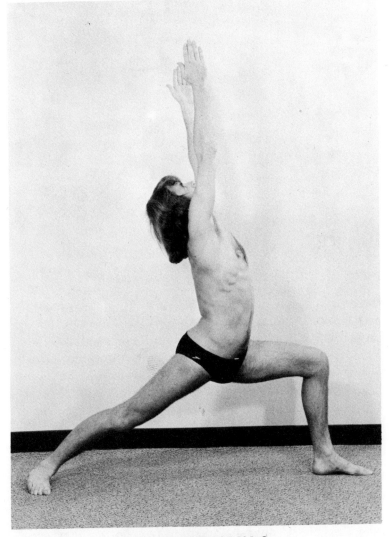

VIRAHABDRASANA 2

I have tried to show the action of this pose by exaggerating
it a little. The feet are the same distance apart as the poses on
the facing pages. The forward leg is bent at a right angle, and
the back leg is straight. The body is twisted so that it faces
forward, as shown by the position of the arms. The idea is to
bring the straight leg side of the body forward. Do both sides
in each of these first four standing poses.

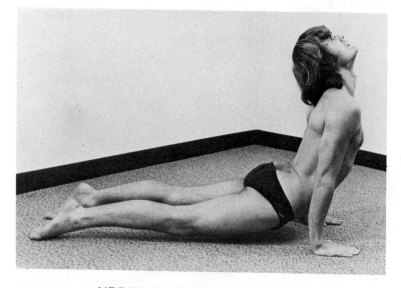

URDHVA MUKHA SHVANASANA

These two poses go together. The names mean " head up dog
pose" and "head down dog pose."
Lie face down, feet about 12 inches apart and hands by the
shoulders as if about to do a push up. Straighten the arms,
lock the elbows and let the body hang down from the shoulders. Bring the hips towards the wrists, dragging the feet on
the ground as you do so. Keep the kneecaps tightened and off
the ground. Tighten the buttocks, arch the head back, and
try to look further behind over your head by slowly increasing the backbend, working with the breath.

Note that the head and neck are not sunk in between the
shoulders but rather extended up so as to create space between the ear lobes and the shoulders. When you first try
the pose, hold it only for a breath or two, but as the edges of
your endurance move out, hold it for half a minute to a minute, or even longer. Whatever turns you on.

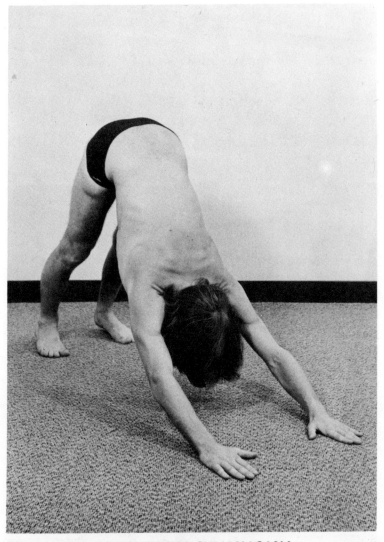

ADHO MUKHA SHVANASANA

To move from this pose to the "head down dog," turn the
toes under, push the buttocks up and back, and try to straight-
en the arms.   Adjust the feet so that the heels are a little off
the ground. While holding the pose, try to push the heels to
the ground and to lift the buttocks higher. Work to lengthen
the spine, all the way from the tailbone to the top of the head.
You can get the feel of lengthening the spine by trying to
push the lower back in. As in all these poses, breathe deeply
and evenly.

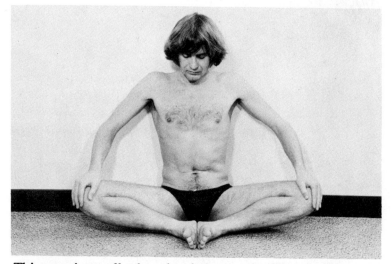

This pose is usually done by sitting on the floor, holding
the feet as shown in the bottom photo, and pulling the
heels in close to the genitals. Then you try to get the knees
down to the floor as you pull up on your hands. Keep
the spine straight and the shoulders pulled back.

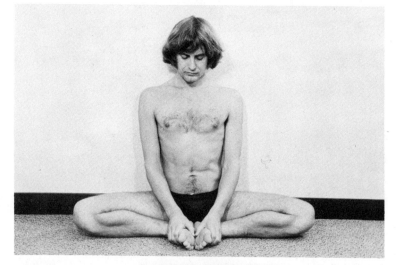

BADDHA KONASANA

I prefer to do this pose with my back to a wall so that I can
hold it for several minutes in complete relaxation. When you
start, you might find the knees way up off the ground. The
idea is to explore your tightness as you stretch towards the
final position.

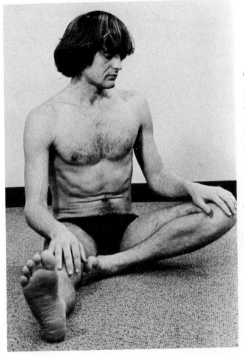

The knee work shown here
is not a yoga pose as such,
but rather a way of loosen-
ing the knee and hip joints
in preparation for the Lotus
pose shown on page 73.
The knees are very delicate
joints, which is why they are
so vulnerable to athletic injuries. If you work with them
carefully, you can improve
their flexibility and resistance to injury, but if you force
them, you'll end up hurting
yourself. Be very cautious
and aware as you work.

Bring the sole of one foot up
against the inner thigh of the
outstretched leg, with the
heel as close to the genitals
as possible. At first, the
bent knee will probably be
well off the ground. Rest
the hand on the knee and
gently (very gently) coax it
down. Work with the breath
as described in the last chapter.

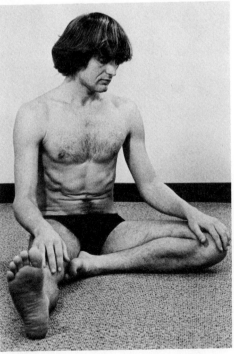

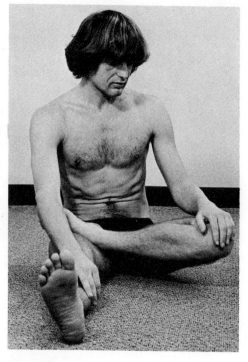

The next step is to work the knee down to the floor when the foot is resting up on the thigh. As you bring the foot up to the thigh, try very gently to push the heel into the navel. Rest the foot on the thigh with the heel touching the abdominal wall if you can manage it without forcing.

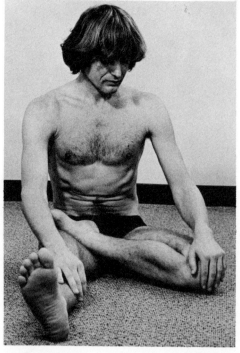

If you find one knee is tighter than the other, spend more time with it until they match up. (This may take years.) In yoga, you quickly discover that the left and right sides of the body are rarely in balance. We do not notice the imbalance, but it reduces the efficiency of our movement and is thus an energy drain.

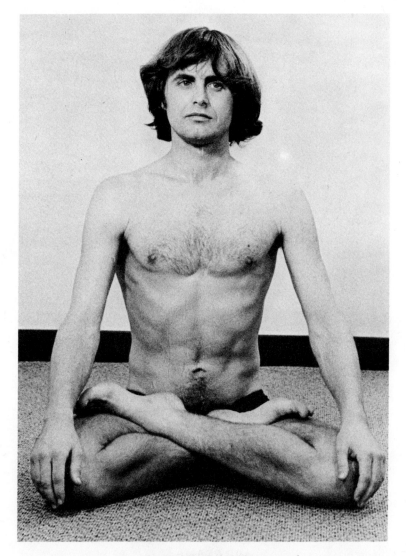

PADMASANA (The Lotus)

Working the knees will gradually increase their flexibility.
You may never be able to do the lotus pose, but that in no
way reduces the value of the knee work. However, if you
do get loose enough to sit this way, it will give you a remark-
ably economical way to make your legs more resilient, since
you have to sit much of the day anyway. It doesn't make
any difference which foot goes up on the thigh first, but be
sure to equalize the time so as not to create imbalance.

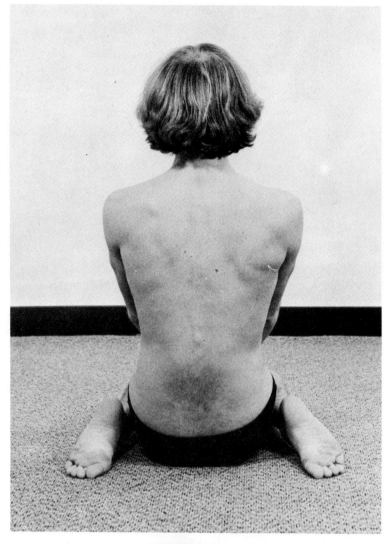

VIRASANA

If you look closely at the way the legs are folded in the knee
work shown on the preceeding pages, you'll notice that the
lower leg is turned in towards the other leg. To work the
knees only in this way is to invite muscular imbalance, so be
sure to spend equal time with this pose, which turns the lower
leg out away from the other leg. Keep the knees together and
carefully lower yourself down to sit on the floor between the
feet. Until you can sit on the floor, put enough cushions under
your buttocks to enable you to sit comfortably.

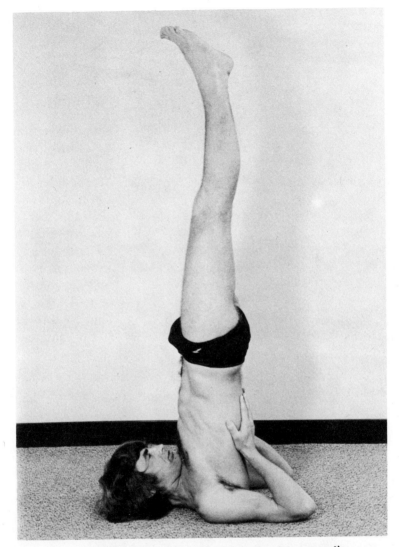

SARVANGASANA (The shoulder stand)

Lie on your back with the legs stretched out. First lift the legs up to vertical, keeping them straight if possible, then lift the whole body up into a straight line. It is easier to position the body correctly if you get the hands close to the floor. Keep the legs straight and position the big toes so that they are directly above the eyes. Breathe deeply and evenly. At first, you might stay in the pose for a few breaths. Later, you can hold it from five to ten minutes. It promotes deep relaxation.

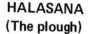

HALASANA
(The plough)

Keep the back as
flat as possible, as
if you were still in
the shoulder stand.
Get the elbows as
close together as
you can. Stay in
the pose for just
a breath or two at
first. As you get
more flexible, ex-
tend the time up
to five minutes.

This pose is a con-
tinuation of the
shoulder stand.
Keeping the legs
straight, let them
come down to
the floor. Don't
force them down.
Let them hang.
Eventually gra-
vity will pull them
down.

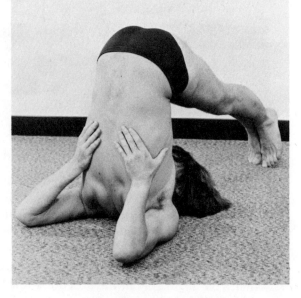

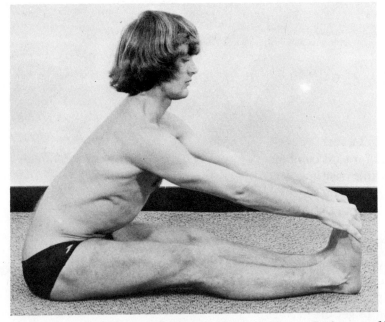

Reach only as far as you comfortably can. If you find yourself
on the edge of your stretch when you are holding your legs just
below your knees, that's where you should stay and play.

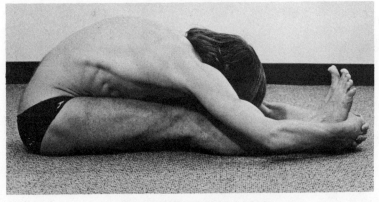

PASCHIMOTTANASANA

A whole lot of stretching going on. When you get this far down,
you can extend the spine more by widening the elbows. You
can increase the stretch on the backs of the legs by moving the
hands up to the balls of the feet , pushing the heels away from
your sitting bones, pressing the backs of the knees into the
floor, and pulling back on your hands.

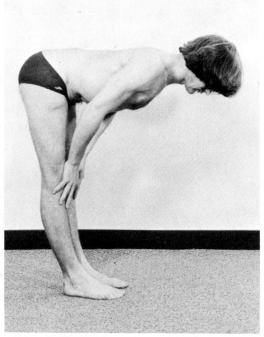

To get a feel for correct forward bending, try this position. Keep the knees locked by pulling up on the knee caps. Try to lift the sitting bones up higher and to extend the spine. To extend the spine, work to flatten the back and to get the head as far away from the sitting bones as possible.

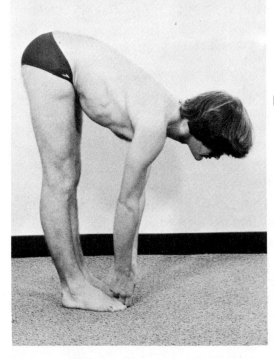

PADANGUSHTHASANA

As you get more flexible, move your hands down your legs until you can secure a hold on your big toes between your first two fingers and your thumbs. Always work to extend the spine. Try to push in the lower back so as to get the belly in contact with the upper thighs.

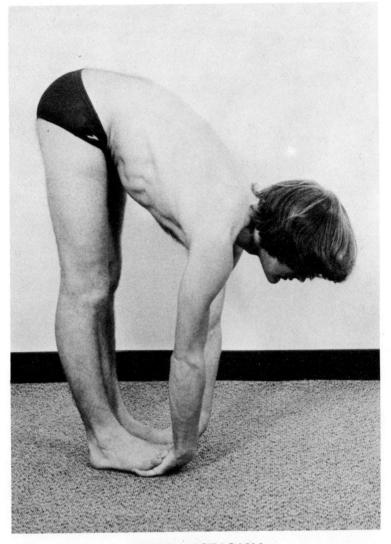

PADA HASTASANA

When you're comfortable holding on to the big toes, you can
try pushing your hands under the balls of your feet. If you
look closely at the way my back is bending, you will notice a
point, at the end of the dark hair on my lower back, where
the bend breaks. The lower back is flat to that point, and
the back bends from there. You will probably discover something similar in your own back. Work to flatten this "break."
It helps to drop the head so that the spine has an even curve
up to the base of the skull.

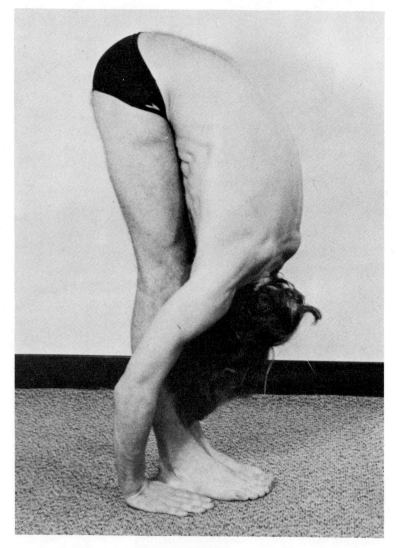

UTTANASANA

When you get quite loose, you will be able to put the palms
flat on the floor and press the front of the body against the
thighs. The body and the thighs should come together like
the blades of a pair of scissors—rotating from the hip joint,
the belly should make contact, then the chest, and finally the
head can be buried between the legs.

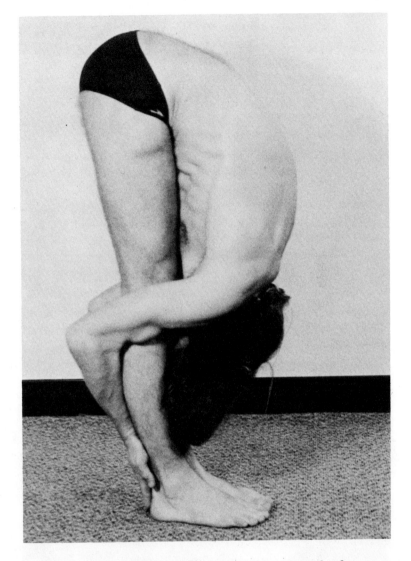

I have found it easier to work in this pose when the forearms are tucked in behind the calves. The hamstring stretch is intensified by trying to push the sitting bones up higher, away from the heels, and the spine is lengthened further by trying to move the head closer to the feet with each breath. An important part of both warm-up and cool-down, this pose can also be used between tempo runs in a speed workout.

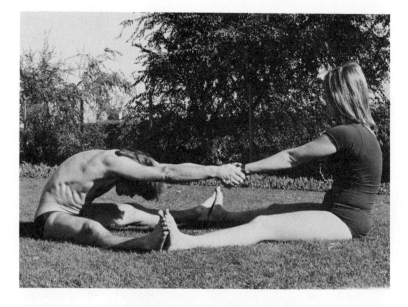

Yoga at noon. Few are fortunate enough to have a lawn outside the office for yoga practice, but everyone can find a small
space somewhere.   If you don't mind being stared at, you can
do yoga stretches right by your desk at work or at school.
Stretching brings a feeling of lightness and energy. It's a better
way of spending the lunch hour than eating, especially if you
can get together with a friend.

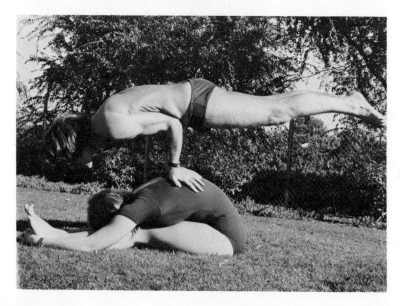

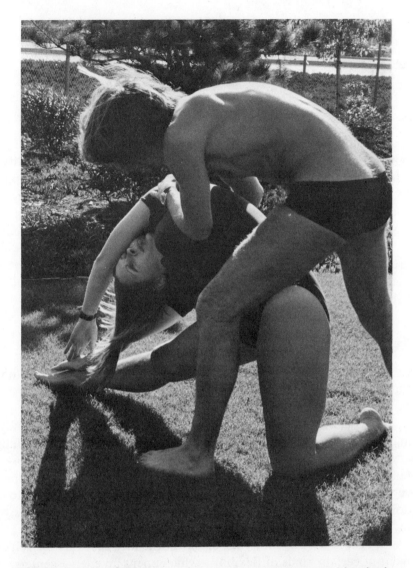

Sue Turner in Parighasana. The adjustment I am making is similar to the adjustment I would be making in teaching the triangle pose. The upper shoulder is being coaxed back and the lower shoulder coaxed forward, thus increasing the stretch on her left side. Although essentially a solitary pursuit, yoga has many moods, including the mood of relaxed play.

14 Playing the Edges

I was sitting on the floor, gingerly testing a sore hamstring. I had hurt it the night before in my eagerness to be at a peak of flexibility for a long-awaited yoga workshop. The teacher, Joel Kramer, was reputed to be one of the most adept hatha yogis in the world. Considering the focus of his discussion, it was very timely for me. While listening to him I was aware of the sore leg, and that I had started yoga to *avoid* injuries.

As he began his presentation, I immediately liked him. He looked around the room as he spoke. His natural and open eye contact made me feel part of a personal conversation with him rather than a student listening to a teacher.

"I would like to introduce you to a way of doing yoga that may be different from what you are used to," he said.

"In order to be sure that yoga does not become mere calisthenics, there must be a certain quality of awareness, of mind. Without this, there is no yoga. The focal point is not the gaining of any ends or results, but rather the quality of awareness in the doing."

I thought about the focal point of my yoga practice since studying with Iyengar and Rishi. Although the sensuality of the stretching was still there, the structure of the asanas had become more important. I had not wanted to admit it to myself, but I had been feeling very discouraged by the great gulf between what I was supposed to be doing with my body and what I was capable of doing. Sometimes, my practice had felt like work instead of play.

"People starting into yoga often get the idea that it is the achievement of certain kinds of flexibility which opens up energy centers. And that is true, to an extent. For me, flexibility comes only as a by-product of exploring areas of tightness. Ambition tends to make us tighter. Striving for flexibility can bring flexibility to a certain degree, but in the long run it is detrimental to the total well-being of the person. As soon as we drop the ambition and get into exploring our tightness, the conflict between what we are and what we want to be dissolves, and that brings a physiological relaxation."

I thought back to my racing ambitions, and the havoc they had wrought in my life. Yoga had somehow seemed inherently safe, so

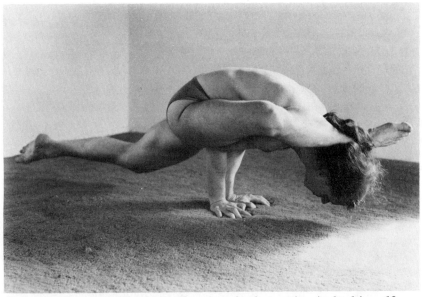

Joel Kramer is an exceptionally adept hatha yogi.   As he himself points out, there is nothing magical about the degree of flexibility he has attained.   When he started, the limits of his stretch were like the typical distance runner's.   He couldn't even come close to touching his toes.   Now, he needs advanced stretches to play his edges. (Above, Hal Friedman photo, below, Jules Kanarek photo)

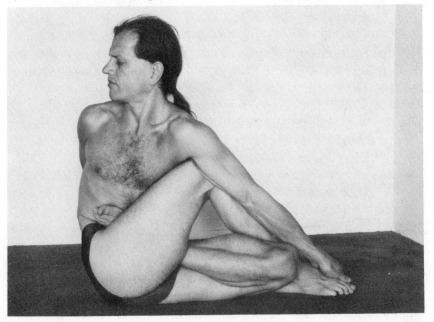

totally out of contact with the competitive spirit that it was a guardian against the excesses of ambition. Now I wasn't so sure about that any more. In all honesty, I had to admit that I had brought the competitive spirit into striving for perfection in the asanas. In spite of warnings from Iyengar and Rishi, I was doing my yoga with a striving mind instead of a receptive body.

"If you approach your yoga as a way of tuning into your body/ mind feedback system, you can very quickly learn to be your own teacher. Teachers come and teachers go, but fundamentally one is always with oneself. You must not accept me as an authority just because I have a certain way with words and certain levels of flexibility. Take what you can from my presentation to open up doors for your own inner exploration. You are never really in touch with yoga until you learn to do it on your own. Teachers are useful guideposts, but if you accept a teacher as an authority and obey blindly, that puts you out of touch with yourself."

I knew what he said was fundamentally true. For many months now, I had been going to Felicity's class or to a teacher training session at least once a week. Regular feedback from a teacher kept my practice from becoming sloppy. There seemed to be more to learn all the time, a steady progression into ever finer precision of structural adjustment. But in spite of these advantages, I much preferred practicing yoga alone, choosing my own pace and my own sequence of asanas. I knew that outside guidance had helped me tremendously, but perhaps I was now ready for more independence.

"In my yoga, the breath is the controlling factor, the inhalations and the exhalations. Beginners usually try to do the asanas with the mind. They have in mind an image of the positions they want to get their bodies into, and they try to force it."

How well that described my own beginnings with Hittleman's book! I recalled the agony I had senselessly endured in trying to reach what I thought was the proper body position.

"When the mind is controlling, there is always a gap between what you are doing and what you want to be doing. The mind has an image of the perfected position, or a memory of yesterday's levels of flexibility or whatever. And it finds the gap between the image and the reality disturbing. It gets anxious, and that anxiety is physical— a bind in the tissue, a blockage of energy.

"If you allow the breath to be the controlling factor, there is no gap. Then there is a total movement of energy which is extraordinarily efficient. And the energy is not dissipated in the push to get past the edges of your tightness, but it enters into the exploration of the edges.

"When you are working in an asana, your edges, or limits, reveal themselves to you in the sensations of stretch in the muscles and joints. You have to tune into body/mind feedback to play the edges with awareness. Playing your edges elicits a quality of attention which places you in the living instant. This is the essence of yoga."

I tried to remember the quality of awareness in my recent practice, but I couldn't really be sure about it. I was not even sure if last night's practice had been alive and aware. My sore hamstring suggested that striving for perfection had deadened it.

"Yoga is self-exploration. It's a way of learning about yourself. Learning and exploring take energy. If while actually doing yoga you are comparing yourself with others, or with your idea of the perfect posture, or with anything else, the energy you devote to comparison is lost from yoga."

"We have been conditioned to be accomplishment oriented," Kramer continued. "But to be accomplishment oriented in yoga is to remove the energy from the process. It's the doing of the yoga that's got to turn you on. If achieving certain levels of flexibility turns you on, then you're going to find yourself aiming at them. The paradox is that the more you are interested in the goals, and the less in the doing, the less accomplishments come. The less you are interested in them, the more they come."

I thought back to my running, and how I had amazed myself in racing time after time. I remembered how easy running, for the sheer joy of it, had led to marathon times that I simply couldn't believe. And I remembered how everything had turned sour: when, having tasted success as an accidental by-product of doing something I loved, I began to get greedy for more, and to grasp for it.

"For me, the doing of yoga is learning how really to tune into the feedbacks, to the energy. In a very real sense, yoga for me is play. It is playing with oneself in a very intimate and direct way. And, as is the case with all play, yoga doesn't take any effort. This might be hard to grasp at first, but you see it whenever you watch a child playing. A child at play expends an enormous amount of energy, but no effort. Yoga is adult play, and, like child's play, it involves a great amount of energy, but no effort."

I thought back to my best marathon, and the uncanny feeling of just sitting back for a free ride and paying attention simply to keeping the running body in trim. I spent all my energy in that race. I was exhausted when I crossed the finish line. But the energy seemed to flow through me. All I had to do was use it economically. I didn't have to strive to generate it. It came by itself; the race situation called it out.

"Whenever you force yourself, you're forcing yourself towards something—a goal, an end, a result. The end becomes the focal point of attention. You get trapped in pushing yourself towards that end, whether it be a completed posture, releasing a bind in the body, or, more remotely, the ideas you have about self-improvement, higher consciousness or enlightenment."

I added to myself "or the desire to run a sub-2:30 marathon." Everything that Kramer was saying about yoga applied directly to my running experience. I had to admit that I had not fully learned the lesson. My sore hamstring was painful proof that I was still attached to striving for goals.

"The effort of goal striving actually works against us, because it tightens us. As we try to become something, that very effort actually clamps the tissue. Part of the learning in yoga is learning about this, tuning in to when the mind and body are doing this. The fact of the matter is that most of us are ambitious, and when we first begin to do yoga, we bring that ambition to our yoga. I am not saying one should try to get rid of ambition, for that is just another ambition. What I am saying is that when one becomes alert to the nature of ambition, one sees its destructive qualities and its binding nature. When one sees this clearly, ambition becomes less interesting. Yoga can teach you about this in a very intimate way, both physically and psychologically.

If this were all that yoga had to offer, I thought, it would be more than enough to recommend it to any athlete. With this kind of sensitivity and awareness, sport becomes play. All energy and no effort. Tuning in to how effort tightens the tissues can work on a day to day training basis, or on a stride by stride racing basis. When effort comes in, the joyful play of energy goes out. When force is applied to the body, it becomes dull.

What Kramer had to say about energy and effort reinforced my own hard-won insights about the racing obsession. And as he discussed the psychological aspects of yoga, he expressed the same ideas that had occurred to me when I discovered Wilhelm Reich and Ida Rolf.

"There's nothing mysterious about tightening. It's something you do to yourself, over the years. All the daily irritations, frustrations and anxieties accumulate in the muscles, and, as you condition yourself with habits, they also get etched into the body.

In attaining this kind of flexibility, you work out tightness in the mind as well as tightness in the body. (Hal Friedman photo)

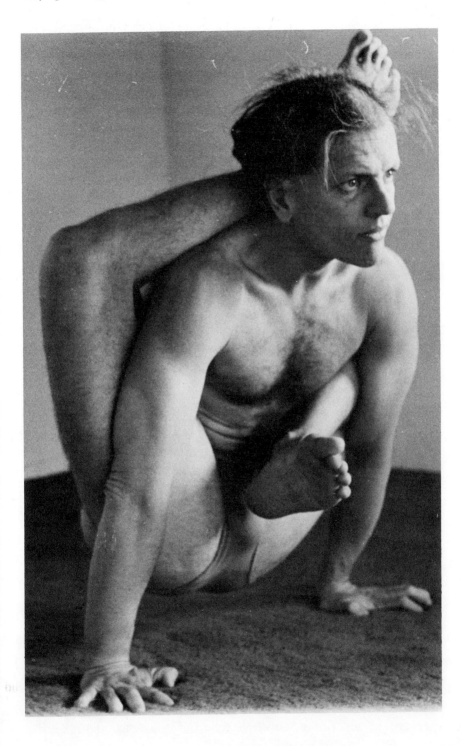

"Most of us take our psychological problems, put impressive sounding labels on them, and in one way or another forget about them or make them unreachable. But if there is a problem in me, it is *in* me, in the nerves, in the glands, in the response repertoire of the body. To learn about this is to see that the division between the mind and the body is not real. The mind and body are not two separate entities, but rather two aspects of one energy system.

"The conditionings, the traumas, the hang-ups, call them what you will, actually live in you. They don't live in a name or in a psychology book, but right in the tissues, in the nerves, in the musculature, in the way the body holds itself. You really learn about this in yoga."

I thought back to the emotional patterns touched off by certain asanas, and I wondered how much of my growing sense of decisiveness and clarity was due to the release of emotional problems stored up in tight muscles. I also thought forward, and wondered where this release was going to take me.

Every day brought new surprises. My life already seemed to be going wildly and beautifully out of control. The more I shrugged off ideas about how I *should* feel and act, the more I expressed how I actually *did* feel, the more I appreciated the free flow of spontaneity and openness.

Kramer's ideas about the spiritual aspect of yoga also struck a responsive chord in me. The spiritual aspect had always made me a little uncomfortable, because I couldn't really get into it. I couldn't meditate, or at least I couldn't do what I had been led to believe was meditation. So I got deeply into my body. When people asked me if I meditated, I told them, "Not in the usual sense, but I do meditate in the asanas. For me, a heavy three-hour session is a three-hour meditation on the body."

But I got the impression that no one was buying my version of meditation. It just wasn't "spiritual" enough. I found myself getting defensive about it. When people kidded me about how much I was into my body, I'd just laugh and say, "Why not? It's the only home I have."

"There is a great deal of confusion about spirituality in yoga," said Kramer. "Most people who consider themselves spiritual seekers are looking for greater depth of experience, more profound insights, higher realms of consciousness. In short, they want deeper, richer, and if possible, longer lasting experiences. After we have collected many of the so-called mundane experiences, like college, psychotherapy, groups, sex, drugs, the whole gamut of it, we hear about spirituality and we say, 'That's for me!' Spirituality is painted as the experience to end all experiences. That's quite enticing, you know. But seeking more experience is just another self-centered activity, no matter how profound or spiritual the experience is said to be. Spirituality comes in a different way from seeking greater depth of experience.

"If you read the great spiritual books of the world, you find they all say the same thing. There's really only one place to look, and that's within, within you. For the universe displays itself within you. And nobody can do that for you. Nobody can guide you as deeply within yourself as you can. Nobody has that inner touch. Nobody can play your edges for you.

"Yoga, spiritually, mentally and physically, is a way of playing with the edges or frontiers of one's being. Real adeptness in yoga lies in how awarely one plays with the edges. In the body itself you experience your edge as a special quality of sensation, generally right before pain. It is difficult to describe since it is a non-verbal experience, but it is not difficult to discover for yourself. The feeling of energy is the key. By the feeling of pain, I mean discomfort which the mind seeks to escape. Thus, if you push past your edge into pain, attention has been removed from yoga."

"Many of us approach yoga like puritans," he said. "We go under the saying 'no pain, no gain.' The pain makes us feel that we are doing something good to ourselves. But real yoga is not a play with pain. Pain blocks the necessary quality of attention. If you try to ignore it, then you are operating out of greed or ambition. Of course, you can learn from that, because that's where you pull muscles. You see, greed lives with you for a while."

Yes, greed was still living with me. I thought back to the physical breakdown following my long bout of overtraining. Greed lived with me for months after that. Greed for goals is basically the same, in yoga and running.

"If your images of what is structurally correct become goals you strive for, they can be destructive. This is a difficult point, so please don't jump to conclusions about what I mean. Structures can be useful toys to play with. The danger comes when the toy becomes the final authority so that one forces oneself to the structure, ignoring one's edges. This is the stuff of violence.

"To get into any asana is to play with structure, to some extent. Structures tune you into the feedback networks. To be involved with hatha yoga is to be involved with structures. The destructive element comes in when the structure becomes the goal that you're shooting for.

"Take the image of correct structure in the headstand, for instance. To try to force yourself into the correct image is to lose the quality of exploration. Rather than using an image, I work with the muscles and bones, and let them be the guide through feedback. The spine should be straight in the headstand, not because anyone says so, but because your body tells you so.

"The body tells you through feedback. I tune into the pressures on the spine. I tune into the point of contact on my head. I play with gravity as it works through my body. When my headstand is weightless, with no strain, then I know it is right. Only through the process of internal play, a continuous readjusting, does the body get a chance to tell you that the spine is straight.

"A natural tendency of mind is to get oriented towards results, goals. I don't think you should resist this tendency, because resistance is just another goal. Remain aware of it, and through that quality of awareness you leave yourself malleable.

"For me, the interest is in the inner feel of how the musculature works and where the greatest efficiency in the stretch is. If your interest is the efficiency of the stretch at the instant, then really there isn't any goal involved. And when your interest is in the maximum efficiency of stretch, automatically the proper structures come. In fact, this is how the structure of the asanas evolved over the centuries."

I translated this into running terms. If your interest is in the running itself ("On action alone by thy interest"), on the rhythm of the arms and legs, the body carriage, the breathing, then you are running in the living instant rather than in some future race.

"One of the little tricks of yoga is generally to do your weak side first. You might find, for instance, that your triangle pose is much better on the left side than the right. If you do the strong side first, you have an unconscious tendency to try forcing the weak side up to the same standards of accomplishment. So you push yourself, and as you push, the muscles clamp down.

"If you do the weak side first, it is easier to devote more energy to it. You get frustrated when you do it after the strong side, and you tend to spend less time with it. Moreover, if you do your weak side first, you can always do it again after you have done your strong side, to bring a balance.

"We are tempted to go for our strong side because we have been conditioned to go for accomplishment. It is un-American not to go for accomplishment, but it is also un-Indian and un-Chinese too. It's no different anywhere. Accomplishment is the carrot we dangle in front of ourselves.

"But if you strive for accomplishment, then you tend to ignore pain. Pain can mean many things, but no matter what it means, you risk pulling muscles if you try to push past it. You can take risks if you want to, but why not use the pain as a sign that your attention is wandering and your body is complaining. Then you can back off and begin to play with it.

"In some ways it's like a flirtation. It's like flirting with the edges of oneself. And that flirtation must have a quality of attention if it is to open up the tissues. If I'm not right here—now, if I'm off in some image of what I want or in stoic endurance of the pain, then I cut myself off from the exploration which is yoga.

"Yoga is learning to play with feeling. Yoga *is* feeling. Although the books don't write it up this way, it is probably the most sensual activity you can engage in.

"Pain can turn yoga into a chore or a discipline in the destructive meaning of the word. Destructive discipline is doing stuff you really don't want to but think you should because you're hungry for the goal it's supposed to take you to. I think this kind of discipline is a form of self-abuse.

"The root meaning of discipline is to learn. Simply to learn. To be truly disciplined is to be totally involved in learning. If your yoga becomes a chore or a play in pain rather than an exploration, then you're going to find yourself not doing it.

"I'm not interested in yoga as a chore. I'm interested in it as a mode of play, a really intimate way of playing with oneself. The whole secret of yoga is just doing it for the sake of doing it. No goals, no objectives, no gains, no losses. Once the mind gets into that perspective, there is an automatic release of tension.

"It's really very simple. You've just got to dig it. If you don't dig it, it doesn't happen. That's the way it is. You've got to love doing it. And by love I mean a quality of passion, a quality of abandonment. It is the doing of it that is the heart of yoga."

Kramer began to prepare for a demonstration of postures. As he unbuttoned his shirt, he continued to speak.

"What you will see is not the way I work when I am alone. Usually, I stay with each pose longer, and my breathing becomes much deeper and slower. There is nothing magical about the degree of flexibility I have attained. It came naturally as I contined to play the edges over the years. As the edges got further out, I had to start using these advanced and intricate poses. The easy poses simply were nowhere near my edge anymore.

"One of the secrets of continued exploration, especially as you get very flexible, is always to spend a few breaths away from the edge. Even though you know you have the flexibility to hit it hard, don't. Begin at the beginning every day; approach the edge slowly, with the breath."

And with this Kramer cut short his introductory remarks. As he took off his shirt and pants, he seemed already to be internalizing, to be withdrawing into his body awareness. He was wearing brief swim trunks, and although his muscles were not bulky they were extraordinarily well defined. His movements had that relaxed fluidity that I have come to associate with all people who have been into hatha yoga for some time. He began with the headstand, breathing deeply and evenly as he moved into it. From the basic headstand, he moved through a cycle of variations, twisting his body to one side and the other, then folding his legs into the lotus pose and twisting again.

His breath grew steadily deeper, and it became obvious what he meant when he said that he let the breath control rather than the brain. It was his breathing that moved him. When twisting, for instance, he would go a little distance on the exhalation, hold on the inhalation, then move deeper into the twist on the next exhalation.

Using this method, he began to do fantastic things with his body, working into poses that I had only seen photos of up till that time. There was a quality of great power and grace in his every movement. He executed the most difficult and intricate poses with consummate ease. As I watched him, I sensed that he was letting himself be moved, rather than exerting the effort to control. Seeing his demonstration tied it all together for me.

For Further Exploration

Articles by Ian Jackson

"To Eat or Not to Eat"—Chapter 1 of *The Runner's Diet* (RMB No. 14).
"Yoga: Balancing the Imbalance"—*Nordic World*, November, 1973.
"Yoga for the Runner"—*Exercises for Runners* (RMB No. 29).
"The Ski-less Summer: Yoga"—*Nordic World*, July, 1974.
"Make Everything Count"—*Aquatic World*, November, 1973.
"Get Out of the Way"—*Bike World*, February, 1974.
"The Root of All Training"—*Runner's World*, May, 1973.
"The Fun Way of Gutting It Out"—*Runner's World*, November, 1974.
"Yoga for the Gymnast?"—*Gymnastics World*, January, 1975.
All Sports Yoga Routine—pamphlet included free on request with all book orders from the World Publications sports books catalog.
"Yogarobic Running" in Chapter 10 of *The Complete Runner*.

Recommended Reading

The Conditioning of Distance Runners, by Tom Osler.
Long Slow Distance: The Humane Way to Train, by Joe Henderson.
The Complete Runner, by the editors of *Runner's World*.
Guide to Distance Running, edited by Bob Anderson and Joe Henderson.
The Nightmare of Success, by Bill Ruzicka.
Food for Fitness, from the editorial staff of World Publications.
Natural Hygiene, by Herbert Shelton.
Health for the Millions, by Herbert Shelton.
Fasting for Renewal of Life, by Herbert Shelton.
The Hygienic System, vol. 3 (the definitive work on fasting), by Herbert Shelton.
Food Combining Made Easy, by Herbert Shelton.
Superior Nutrition, by Herbert Shelton.
Health is Your Birthright, by Are Waerland.
Exercises for Runners, from the editorial staff of *Runner's World*.
Yoga Self-Taught, by Andre Van Lysebeth.
Light on Yoga, by B. K. S. Iyengar.
The Passionate Mind, by Joe Kramer. (In bookstores or by mail for $4.50 from Joel Kramer, Box 363, Bolinas, CA 94924. Write to the same address for information on yoga lecture/demonstrations, seminars and workshops.)

If you cannot find the books you want at your local bookstore, write for the World Publications Catalogue, P.O. Box 366, Mountain View, CA 94040.

Yoga, Iyengar Style—for information on teachers trained in the Iyengar method, write California Yoga Teachers' Association, 1736 Ninth Ave., San Francisco, CA 94122. (415) 566-4100.

Rolfing—for general information and a nationwide listing of trained and certified Rolfers, write Richard A. Stenstadvold, Executive Director, Rolf Institute of Structural Integration, P. O. Box 1868, Boulder, CO 80302.

RUNNER'S WORLD
WORLD
MAGAZINE

Run longer and more gently with **Runner's World,** the magazine for all running enthusiasts.

- Complete coverage of the most interesting and dramatic races.
- In-depth interviews and penetrating personality profiles of the key figures in the sport.
- Running shorts, racing highlights, coming events, news and views.
- Medical advice column from Dr. George Sheehan.
- Each issue is a valuable addition to your running—each is solidly packed with practical, useful, informative articles.

RUNNER'S WORLD MAGAZINE
Post Office Box 366
Mountain View, CA 94040

Please enter my subscription for the following—
_____ Renewal _____ New Subscription
_____ One Year (monthly — 12 issues) $9.50 _____ Two Years $18.00
_____ Three Years $25.50 _____ Five Years $40.00 _____ Ten Years $70.00

NAME_____

ADDRESS_____

CITY/STATE/ZIP_____

For faster service, please enclose payment